Physiological Society Study Guides *Nu*

The control of breathing in man

Physiological Society Study Guides

1 **Acid-base balance**
edited by R. Hainsworth *0 7190 1981 8 (hb) –1982 6 (pb)*

2 **Amino acid transport in animal cells**
edited by D. L. Yudilevich and C. A. R. Boyd *0 7190 2432 3 (hb) –2433 1 (pb)*

3 **The control of breathing in man**
edited by B. J. Whipp *0 7190 2463 3 (hb) –2464 1 (pb)*

Physiological Society Study Guides *Number 3*

The control of breathing in man

Edited by
B. J. Whipp

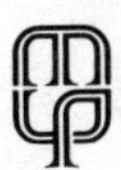

Manchester University Press

Published by Manchester University Press
Oxford Road, Manchester M13 9PL, UK

British Library cataloguing in publication data
The Control of breathing in man. –
(Physiological Society study guides; no. 3).
1. Respiration
I. Whipp, Brian J. II. Series
612′.21 QP121

ISBN 0 7190 2463 3 *hardback*
ISBN 0 7190 2464 1 *paperback*

Typeset in Hong Kong
by Graphicraft Typesetters Ltd., Hong Kong

Printed and bound in Great Britain
by Billing & Sons Limited, Worcester.

Contents

List of contributors vii
Preface viii
Some symbols used in respiratory physiology xi

1 **The control of breathing pattern** 1
- 1.1 Introduction 1
- 1.2 Breath-by-breath variability 2
- 1.3 Changes of breathing pattern with increasing respiratory drive 3
- 1.4 Mechanical factors 8
- 1.5 Neural influences 13
- 1.6 Dynamic changes of breathing pattern 15
- 1.7 The neural drive 21
- 1.8 The work and O_2 cost of breathing 22
- 1.9 A note about measurement 23
- 1.10 Concluding comments 24
- 1.11 Further reading 26

2 **The ventilating responses to hypoxia** 29
- 2.1 Introduction 29
- 2.2 Steady-state characteristics 29
- 2.3 Contribution of the carotid bodies to hypoxic sensitivity 32
- 2.4 Contribution of other mechanisms to hypoxic sensitivity 33
- 2.5 Dynamic response characteristics 38
- 2.6 Modulators of hypoxic sensitivity 39
- 2.7 Methods for assessing hypoxic sensitivity 40
- 2.8 Further reading 41

3 **The ventilatory response to inhaled CO_2** 45
- 3.1 Introduction 45
- 3.2 Steady-state methods 45

3.3 The rebreathing method 47
3.4 Dynamic responses 48
3.5 Measurement of input 50
3.6 Measurement of output 52
3.7 Theoretical and practical problems in performing CO_2 response measurement 53
3.8 Interpretation of changes in slope of the CO_2 response 56
3.9 Central and peripheral chemoreceptors: interaction with hypoxia 58
3.10 The CO_2 response and exercise 60
3.11 Applications in physiology, pharmacology and medicine 62
3.12 Further reading 63

4 **Do oscillations in arterial CO_2 tension provide feed-forward control of ventilation?** 68
4.1 Introduction 68
4.2 Measurement of pH as a reflection of arterial CO_2 tension 69
4.3 The timing effect 70
4.4 Phase relationship and ventilatory control 72
4.5 The role of the carotid body 75
4.6 A possible role in mediating exercise hyperpnoea 78
4.7 Further reading 82

5 **Control of exercise hyperpnoea** 87
5.1 Introduction 87
5.2 Determinants of ventilation 88
5.3 Ventilatory response characteristics 94
5.4 Proposed control mechanisms 103
5.5 Further reading 113

Index 119

List of contributors

Brenda A. Cross Departments of Medicine and Physiology, The Middlesex Hospital Medical School London, U.K.

Andrew R. C. Cummin Department of Medicine I, St. George's Hospital Medical School, London, U.K.

Ebbe S. Petersen University Laboratory of Physiology, Oxford, U.K.

Peter A. Robbins University Laboratory of Physiology, Oxford, U.K.

Kenneth B. Saunders Department of Medicine I, St. George's Hospital Medical School, London, U.K.

Stephen J. G. Semple Department of Medicine, The Middlesex Hospital Medical School, London, U.K.

Susan A. Ward Departments of Anesthesiology and Physiology, UCLA, Los Angeles, U.S.A.

Brian J. Whipp Division of Respiratory Physiology and Medicine, Harbor-UCLA Medical Center, Torrance, U.S.A.

Preface

The Physiological Society's Teaching Symposium on 'The Control of Breathing in Man' had as its main purposes a synthesis of the current areas of investigation which form the frontier of human respiratory control, and consideration of the techniques which are, and are becoming more, available to the investigator so that – when placed in historical context – the presentations would suggest the main directions in which the field appears to be heading.

This book, which grew out of that symposium, retains those goals in addition to having 'the student' as its focus: 'the student', in particular, being the undergraduate studying physiology, either for itself or as part of a related discipline such as the other pre-clinical medical sciences, medicine, engineering and physical education. But physiologists and other biomedical scientists are becoming increasingly aware that the bulk of the pertinent information with regard to a control system lies in its transient or nonsteady-state response behaviour. Consequently, in addition to analysis of the more traditional steady-state responses to a particular ventilatory stressor, inferences which may be drawn from techniques of dynamic forcing and analysis are considered. The authors have exemplary credentials for the task; besides being internationally-recognised experts in the topics of their reviews, they all have currently active research programmes in these areas.

Dr Petersen, Chapter 1 begins by considering how the body selects, from an infinite set of possibilities, the appropriate size and duration of a breath under a variety of conditions and, furthermore, how it partitions that breath into an inspiratory and an expiratory phase; whether the flow of gas which is achieved is under instantaneous or previously determined control; and to what extent the resulting pattern of breathing is optimum, from a mechanical and gas-exchange standpoint.

Drs Ward and Robbins, chapter 2, address the issue of how the body responds to the stress of impaired oxygenation of the blood with respect to the sensors, the interaction with other concurrent stimuli, and analysis of the various tests which are employed to assess the quantify the body's response to these stressors.

Drs Cummin and Saunders, chapter 3, consider the topic of the body's responses to altered levels of carbon dioxide in the body fluids and the physiological mechanisms which constrain changes in the acid–base status of the arterial blood when confronted with an increased load of carbon dioxide: either exogenous, via airway administration or endogenous, via exercise.

Drs Cross and Semple, chapter 4, assess the role of the fluctuating levels of carbon dioxide partial pressure in the arterial blood which results from the cyclic nature of the breath. Inspiration dilutes the carbon dioxide levels in both the lung gas and blood, whereas these levels continue to build up during expiration. Consequently, an oscillation of carbon dioxide partial pressure is transmitted in the arterial blood. The evidence for a rate-of-change component of carbon dioxide ventilatory responsiveness from this fluctuating signal is considered as a means of providing a carbon dioxide-linked mechanism of breathing control which operates independently of changes in the mean level of the signal.

In the final chapter, Dr Whipp presents the dilemma of the control of breathing during exercise: the relative precision with which ventilation is normally adjusted to meet the altered oxygen and carbon dioxide exchange requirements of exercise without appropriate stimuli being evident at sites of chemoreception. He analyses the competing theories – the predominantly neural, the predominantly humoral, and the neuro-humoral – which purport to explain the precision of the control. These theories, however, are often so contradictory that the topic appears to be at the stage where it will (to quote Polonius) 'by misdirections find direction out'.

While every effort has been made to be even-handed in the treatment of controversial areas, the reader must recognise that this book presents five approaches to understanding the control of breathing in man. Any success it may achieve must be considered in the light of how effectively it entices students to the original sources in order to make up their own minds. When they can't and the issues perplex, the laboratory beckons.

Some symbols used in respiratory physiology

Gas phase

Primary symbols

P	pressure
F	fractional concentration (in dry gas)
V	volume
$\dot{V}$	flow (i.e., volume per unit time)
f	breathing frequency
R	respiratory exchange ratio

Secondary symbols

A	alveolar
D	dead space
T	tidal
ET	end-tidal
I	inspiratory
E	expiratory
STPD	standard temperature & pressure, dry (0°C, 760 mmHg)
BTPS	body temperature & pressure, saturated
ATPS	ambient temperature & pressure, saturated

Examples

$P_{\mathrm{ET}}\mathrm{O}_2$	end-tidal partial pressure of oxygen
$P_{\bar{\mathrm{A}}}\mathrm{CO}_2$	mean alveolar partial pressure of carbon dioxide
$F_{\mathrm{I}}\mathrm{O}_2$	inspiratory fractional concentration of oxygen
V_{T}	tidal volume
$\dot{V}_E$	expiratory ventilation

Blood phase

Primary symbols

Q	volume
$\dot{Q}$	flow (i.e., volume per unit time)
S	percentage saturation of hemoglobin with oxygen
C	content of gas

Secondary symbols

a	arterial
c	capillary
v	venous

Examples

$P_{a}CO_2$	arterial partial pressure of carbon dioxide
$P_{\bar{c}}O_2$	mean capillary partial pressure of oxygen
$S_{a}O_2$	arterial oxygen saturation
$C_{\bar{v}}CO_2$	mixed venous content of carbon dioxide

Dot over a symbol indicates a time derivative of the primary variable (e.g., $\dot{V}_E$, $\dot{Q}$); bar over a symbol indicates a mean value of the primary variable (e.g., $P_{\bar{A}}\,CO_2$, $C_{\bar{v}}\,CO_2$)

1

The control of breathing pattern

E. S. Petersen University Laboratory of Physiology, Oxford

1.1 **Introduction**

Breathing is caused by rhythmic contractions of skeletal muscle that are entirely dependent upon intact nervous connections from the medulla through the spinal cord and the phrenic and intercostal nerves. The origin of the phasic impulses, together with their control and coordination with related motor acts such as swallowing and speech, is brought about by networks of neurones in the medulla and pons jointly referred to as the **respiratory centres**. These centres are influenced by chemical factors – PO_2, PCO_2 and pH in arterial blood and brain extracellular fluid – and by a multitude of neural factors. Breathing may also be affected at the spinal cord level by segmental and intersegmental reflexes, while voluntary changes are probably mediated by corticospinal pathways which bypass the respiratory centres. Breathing is thus the product of chemical and neural influences on a network of neurones, motor nerves and muscles – the result being dependent on the mechanical properties of the chest, the lungs and the airways.

The pattern of breathing includes not only the **total minute volume** of ventilation ($\dot{V}$) but also its components, **tidal volume** (V_T) and **frequency** (f) and the *durations of inspiration* and *expiration* (T_I, T_E) as well as the **flow patterns** and the **end-expiratory lung volume** (the **functional residual capacity**, FRC). Interest in the pattern of breathing has arisen in relation to several different aspects of breathing.

(a) *Mechanical work of breathing*: the two major components of the work of breathing, the elastic and resistive work, are known to be influenced differently by breathing pattern, and it has for many years been thought that there might be an 'optimal' setting of tidal volume and frequency at which the total work of breathing was minimal.

(b) The *organisation and operation of the respiratory centres.*

(c) *Gas exchange*: dead-space ventilation is clearly affected by changes in the $V_T \cdot f$ relationship, but in addition the distribution of inspired air in the lungs as well as O_2 uptake and CO_2 elimination are affected by the flow pattern.

1.2 Breath-by-breath variability

Even in a 'regularly' breathing individual, a certain amount of variability in the volume and duration of individual breaths is evident from inspection of a spirometric trace (Figure 1.1). Some twenty years ago, Priban (1963) made the interesting observation that such breath-by-breath changes in the steady state tended to occur in opposite directions, so that a large tidal volume was associated with a low frequency and *vice versa*. Ventilation therefore showed less breath-by-breath variability than either of its two components, V_T and f:

$$\dot{V}\ (\mathrm{l \cdot min^{-1}}) = V_T\ (\mathrm{l}) \times f\ (\mathrm{min^{-1}}) = V_T \times 60/T_{tot}(\mathrm{s}) \quad (1.1)$$

where T_{tot} is breath duration. Priban's findings thus imply a direct proportionality between V_T and T_{tot}, which means that individual breath values for V_T plotted against the corresponding T_{tot} fall along a single, straight iso-ventilation line extrapolating to the origin.

Further studies of this 'Priban hunting' during rest, CO_2 inhalation and exercise (Kay *et al.*, 1975; Newsom Davis & Stagg, 1975) have shown that the breath-by-breath variability – when considered in terms of V_T *versus* either T_I or T_E – exhibits an equally ordered behaviour. Thus, the V_T-T_I-T_E diagram in Figure 1.2 shows that T_I and T_E are both positively correlated with V_T from breath to breath, and can be described by linear relationships which extrapolate to the origin. In a given condition, the **mean inspiratory** and **expiratory flows** (V_T/T_I, V_T/T_E) therefore remain more constant from breath to breath than either the volumes or phase durations.

The implication of such findings is that mean inspiratory flow is

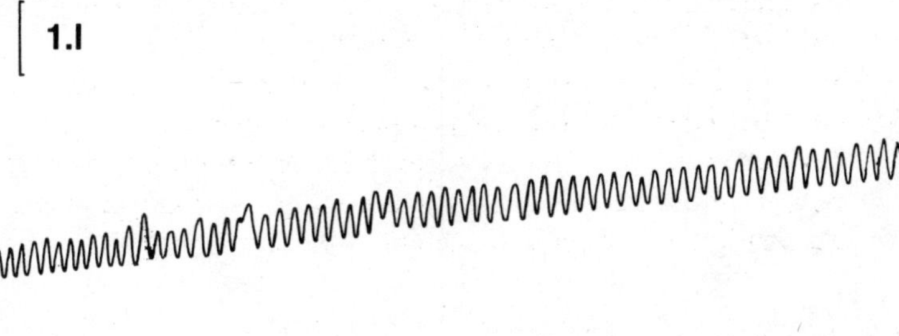

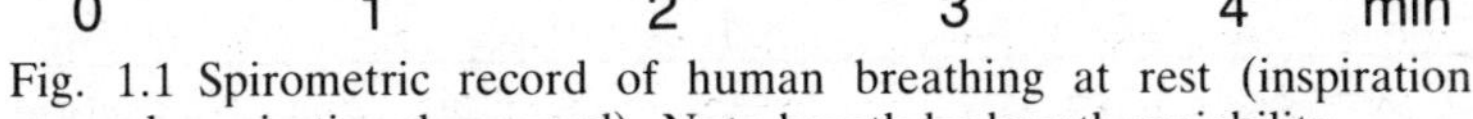

Fig. 1.1 Spirometric record of human breathing at rest (inspiration upward, expiration downward). Note breath-by-breath variability.

set by the prevailing respiratory drive, and that breath-by-breath variations of tidal volume reflect small 'errors' in the mechanisms that determine T_I. Mean expiratory flow may be said to reflect a given recoil pattern, influenced and set by various factors (see below).

1.3 **Changes of breathing pattern with increasing respiratory drive**

The increase in ventilation caused by the inhalation of CO_2-rich and/or O_2-poor gas mixtures or by exercise results characteristically from increases in both tidal volume and frequency. But what has only been appreciated for the last decade or so is that the change in frequency is almost entirely caused by a shortening of mean expiratory time, T_E, while mean inspiratory time, T_I, remains unchanged or only decreases by a small amount. These changes can also be illustrated on the V_T-T_I-T_E diagram (Figure 1.3). The increased ventilation is thus associated with a greater increase of mean expiratory than of mean inspiratory flow on going from a low to a higher ventilation (in this example, from 8 to $30\,l \cdot min^{-1}$); as shown by the steepening of the slope of the broken lines which describe the breath-by-breath V_T-T_I and V_T-T_E variability (cf., Figure 1.2), and thus pass through the mean V_T-T_I and V_T-T_E points (crosses). This observation is of some interest in relation to the often quoted statement that expiration is passive

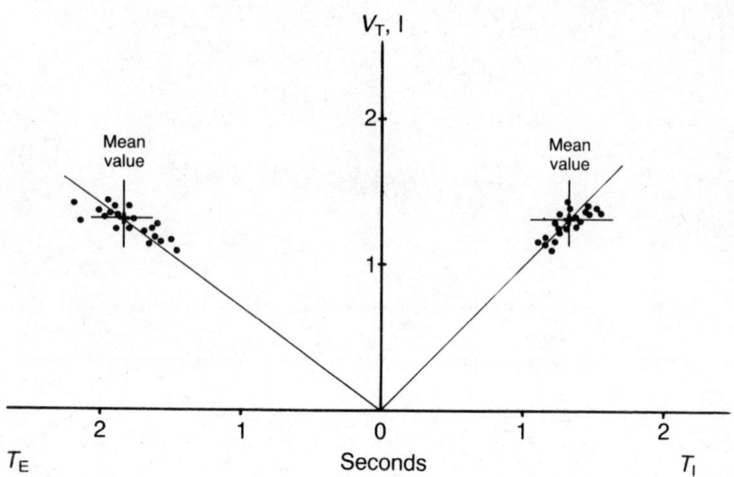

Fig. 1.2 V_T-T_I-T_E diagram indicating the breath-by-breath relationships in man between tidal volume (V_T) and inspiratory duration (T_I) to the right and expiratory duration (T_E) to the left of the origin, for 20 consecutive breaths (+ = mean value) in the steady state of mild hypercapnia ($\dot{V}$ = 25 l · min^{-1}). The corresponding iso-flow lines radiate from the origin through the data points. (Data from Petersen & Vejby-Christensen, 1977.)

and the general agreement from electromyographic (EMG) and other evidence that abdominal muscle activity in man is rarely seen at ventilations less than 40 l · min^{-1}.

Figure 1.3 also shows the mean response of breathing pattern over an extended range of ventilations (heavy lines). For inspiration, this emphasises the relative constancy of T_I at tidal volumes up to some 2–3 l at which stage a **breakpoint** is frequently seen, and above which further rises of V_T are associated with a greater shortening of T_I. The breakpoint has been described as separating a **range 1** with constant or near constant T_I from a **range 2** over which T_I decreases hyperbolically (Gardner, 1977). In the anaesthetised cat and rabbit, range 1 is often absent, and changes of frequency in these animals are therefore less dependent on T_E shortening than they are in man.

Thus, T_I and V_T measured breath-by-breath in a given condition are positively correlated, and the ratio V_T/T_I (the **mean inspiratory flow**) is roughly constant despite variations of T_I and V_T. Mean

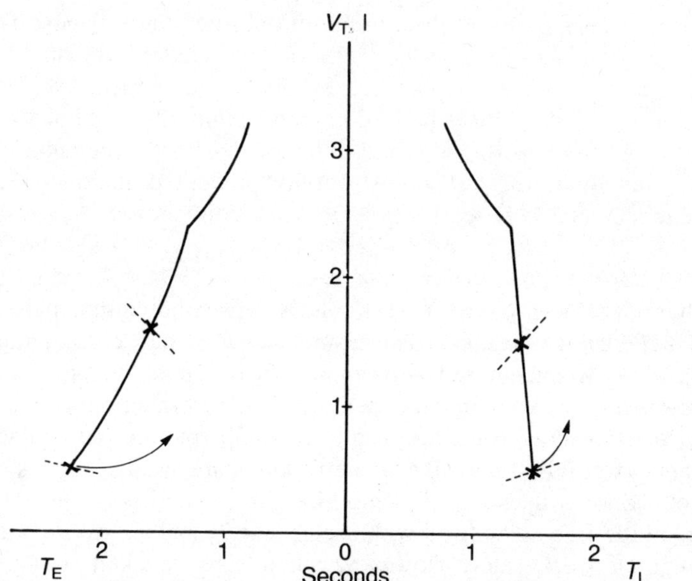

Fig. 1.3 V_T-T_I-T_E diagram indicating the mean V_T-T_I and V_T-T_E relationships in man over a wide range of steady state ventilations; × indicates mean values at $\dot{V}$s of 8 and 30 l · min^{-1} (lower and upper, respectively) together with corresponding iso-flow lines (---) representing the breath-by-breath variation (cf. Figure 1.2). The discontinuities in these steady state relationships separate range 1 over which T_I changes little from range 2 in which a marked T_I shortening is seen. The curved arrows originating from the lower steady state point ($\dot{V}$ = 8 l · min^{-1}) indicate the character of the transient V_T-T_I and V_T-T_E response to a step-increase in respiratory drive: the lengthening of T_I (right) describes the early response to a hypercapnic step, and the shortening of T_E (left) the early response to an hypoxic step.

inspiratory flow may be said to reflect the intensity of the total respiratory drive, which in turn determines the 'central inspiratory activity' (Euler, 1983; see below); T_I is the time taken before the **Hering-Breuer inflation reflex** has reached a sufficient strength to inhibit inspiration. The extended range 1 seen in man has thus been interpreted to imply that the Hering-Breuer reflex is normally weak or even absent, and only activated when breathing encroaches significantly on the inspiratory reserve volume. The absolute V_T at the breakpoint is highly variable between individuals; it appears to be close to about half the vital capacity. The notion of a relatively weak Hering-Breuer reflex in man is in general agreement with earlier reports on the effects of lung inflation in lightly anaesthetised humans. Similarly, vagal block in conscious humans was reported to have no effect on the eupnoeic breathing pattern, but almost totally prevented the increased frequency normally seen with CO_2 inhalation (Guz *et al.*, 1970).

1.3.1 *Hypercapnia, hypoxia and exercise*

There have been reports of differences between breathing pattern in hypercapnia and exercise. Some subjects may entrain their breathing frequency to the frequency of rhythmic movements of the exercising limbs. In our experience, such entrainment is rare in cycling but more common during treadmill running, particularly when external stimuli like a metronome are used. Other subjects consciously adopt a pump-like pattern and maintain their breathing frequency fixed with a constant T_I and T_E over a wide range of work rates. However, when care is taken to avoid external stimuli (e.g. noise from respiratory valves), subjects who are familiar with the procedures change their breathing pattern in the steady state in a remarkably similar way by utilising the same combination of changes of V_T, T_I and T_E in hypercapnia, hypoxia, asphyxia and exercise (a direct isopnoeic comparison of T_I and of T_E at two levels of PCO_2 and PO_2 is shown in Figure 1.4, left).

1.3.2 *Temperature*

One exception to the overall identity of isopnoeic breathing patterns is encountered when breathing is stimulated by a raised body temperature. During hyperthermia, the hyperpnoea induced by hypercapnia and/or hypoxia is characterised by a relatively greater increase of frequency and a correspondingly smaller increase of tidal volume; at any given tidal volume, both T_I and T_E *are shorter*.

Thus, because of the respiratory interactions between CO_2, hypoxia and body temperature, different combinations of these stimuli can induce the same level of ventilatory response and thus allow an isopnoeic comparison of breathing pattern. In Figure 1.4 (left), a comparison can be made of the T_I (top) and T_E (bottom) responses at the same ventilation but for two different values of

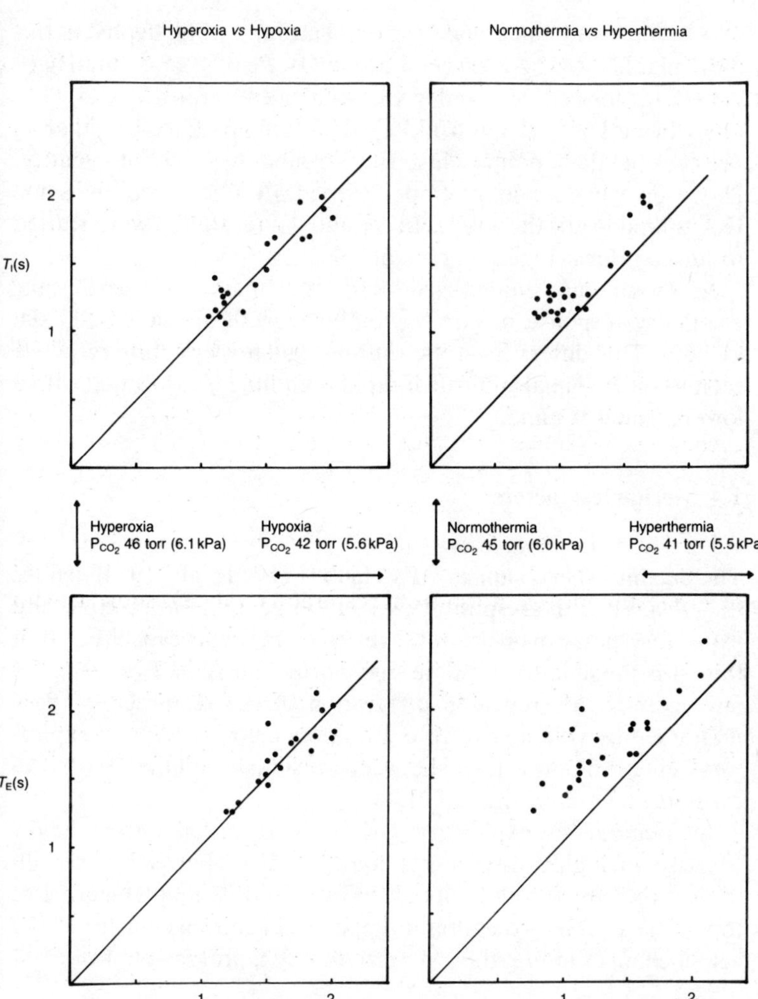

Fig. 1.4 Isopnoeic comparisons. Scattergrams of T_I (upper panels) and T_E (lower panels) in iso-ventilation conditions of increased respiratory drive in man. Left panels: CO_2 in high O_2 *vs* CO_2 in low O_2. Right panels: CO_2 at normal body temperature *vs* CO_2 at a raised body temperature. The left panels show an identical pattern of breathing whether hypoxia is present or not while, in contrast, the right panels show a consistent shortening of both T_I and T_E when hyperthermia is present. (Data from Petersen & Vejby-Christensen, 1977.)

PCO_2, one with and one without accompanying hypoxia: this particular level of hypoxia (end tidal PO_2, $P_{ET}O_2$, ca. 55 mmHg or 7.3 kPa) 'replaced' a 4 mmHg (0.5 kPa) increase in $P_{ET}CO_2$ (i.e. 42 to 46 mmHg or 5.6 to 6.1 kPa). This had no effect on either T_I or T_E; the data points clustering around the line of identity. However, when a rise of temperature (1.4°C) 'replaced' the same CO_2 stimulus, all the isopnoeic T_I and T_E responses were shifted to lower values (Figure 1.4, right).

It should be emphasised that the marked hyperthermic frequency response in man is combined with an increased tidal volume. This differs from the thermoregulatory panting response seen in furry animals, in which rapid breathing is associated with a lowered tidal volume.

1.4 **Mechanical factors**

1.4.1 *Mechanical limitation*

The **maximal flow-volume (MFV) loop** (Fry & Hyatt, 1960) defines the capacity of the respiratory system to generate inspiratory and expiratory flows over the total range of the vital capacity. From this, it is possible to calculate the shortest possible T_I and T_E for any given V_T by repeated integration of the reciprocal of flow multiplied by volume over the total possible range of end-expiratory lung volumes (i.e. between residual volume and vital capacity) (Jensen *et al.*, 1980).

A spontaneous expiratory *FV* curve recorded during heavy exercise in highly fit subjects may actually approach, or even exceed the enveloping limits given by the MFV loop (Figure 1.5, top). The V_T-T_I-T_E diagram in Figure 1.5 (bottom) illustrates the actual changes in breathing pattern during a progressive work test

---

Fig. 1.5 (opposite) Top: flow-volume loops in man for a maximal effort manoeuvre at rest (outer) and for spontaneous breathing during maximal exercise (inner). Bottom: V_T-T_I-T_E diagram indicating (*a*) mean V_T-T_I and V_T-T_E relationships during progressive exercise, with lower break-point separating range 1 from range 2 at a V_T of 31 (cf., Figure 1.3) and a second higher, more marked breakpoint at very high levels of V, and (*b*) the smallest possible T_I and T_E values associated with a particular V_T, as predicted from the maximal effort flow-volume loop and shown by the inner smooth curves. (Data from Jensen *et al.*, 1980.)

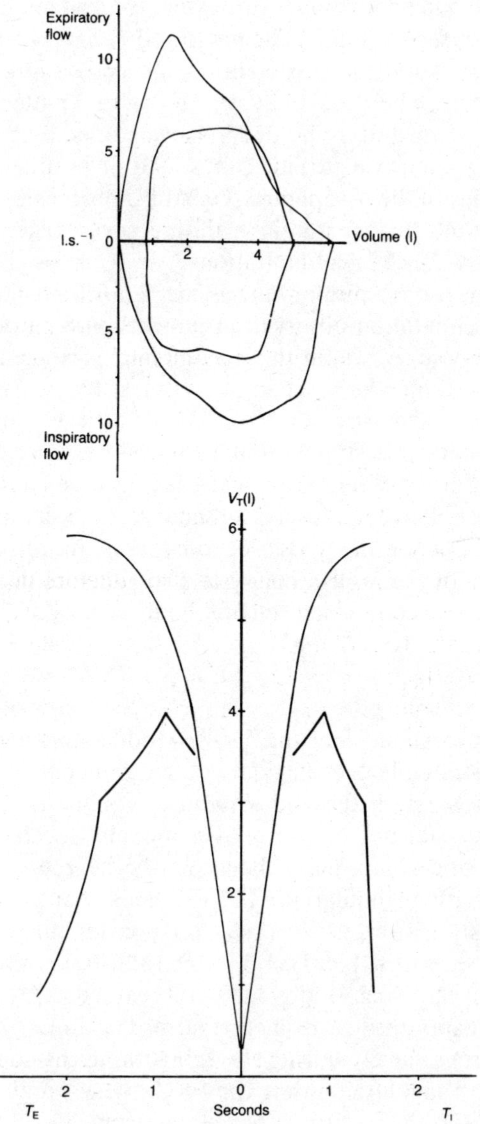
Expiratory
flow
10
5
l.s.⁻¹ 0
2
4
Volume (l)
5
10
Inspiratory
flow
V_T(l)
6
4
2
2
1
0
1
2
T_E
Seconds
T_I

extended to maximum, and the estimated minimal T_I and T_E values (Jensen *et al.*, 1980). The measured T_I and T_E approach the estimated limits at the highest ventilations, and a sudden change in breathing pattern becomes evident. The range 2 pattern of a rising V_T is replaced by a decrease of V_T accompanied by a steeper rise of frequency due to a further shortening of both T_I and T_E. It appears that the central neural control of breathing pattern at these near maximal ventilations during severe exercise can be overridden by mechanical limitations.

Disturbances of respiratory mechanics contribute importantly to the exercise limitation observed in patients with chronic obstructive lung disease, in whom the **maximum expiratory flow-volume** (MEFV) curve may be reached at rest or at low work rates.

The shape and size of the MEFV curve, including its effort-independent portion at lung volumes below ca. 70% of vital capacity, differs between individuals. It is now generally accepted that expiratory flow limitation is a function of the size and the state of the airways, of the cross-sectional area in relation to the distensibility of the walls. Together these factors determine the maximal wave speed, which sets the limit for flow at the so-called choke point (cf., Hyatt, 1983).

1.4.2 *Lung volume*

It will be appreciated that the V_T-T_I-T_E diagrams in Figures 1.2 and 1.3 illustrate changes in tidal volume rather than in absolute lung volume. Only if the end-expiratory volume (FRC) remains constant with changing drive would changes in V_T faithfully reflect changes in lung volume and thence in the degree of pulmonary mechanoreceptor stimulation. If FRC does change, however, a rather grossly distorted V_T-T_I-T_E relationship may result. An example is shown in Figure 1.6, which illustrates the results of experiments in which individuals rebreathed CO_2 through a non-elastic expiratory resistance (Garrard & Lane, 1978). FRC increased progressively during the rebreathing (by some 2 l), and replotting the data after adding the FRC changes to the measured V_T's established the pattern indicated by the heavy, full lines. This pattern was closely similar to that found in control experiments without the resistance, in which FRC did not change (cf., Figure 1.3).

Comparisons of changes in breathing pattern during increasing

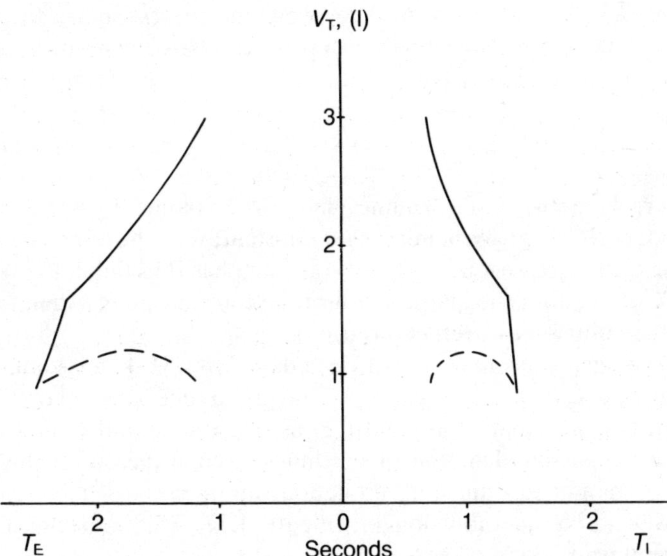

Fig. 1.6 V_T-T_I-T_E diagram indicating mean V_T-T_I and V_T-T_E relationships in man during CO_2 rebreathing with expiratory non-elastic resistance before (----) and after (———) correction of the measured V_T for observed changes in functional residual capacity (i.e. to provide absolute changes in lung volume). (Data from Garrard & Lane, 1978.)

respiratory drive as depicted by the V_T-T_I-T_E diagrams are thus clearly influenced by any changes in FRC that may have taken place. The extent to which this occurs in healthy man during unloaded breathing is not entirely clear. However, both active expiration (which usually becomes evident at ventilations of ca. $40 \text{l} \cdot \text{min}^{-1}$) and changes in the balance between the elastic recoil forces exerted by the lungs and chest wall might affect FRC.

Changes in lung volume with increasing levels of ventilation are unlikely to influence the V_T-T_I-T_E relationship in range 1, but may well affect the V_T at which the breakpoint occurs, the pattern in range 2 and the abrupt changes seen at very high ventilations in exercise (Figure 1.5).

1.4.3 *Expiratory flow*

The driving pressure during a relaxed passive expiration is provided by the **elastic recoil** (P_{el}) of the respiratory system. This pressure is determined by the inspired volume and the **compliance**

($C = \Delta V / \Delta P_{el}$), and is used to overcome the **resistance to flow** (R). The volume-time relationship for a passive expiration may thus be altered by changes of R and/or C (Brody, 1954)

$$V = V_0 \cdot e^{-t/RC} \tag{1.2}$$

where V_0 is the initial volume, and V the volume at time t. The product RC is the **mechanical time constant**, with the dimension of time. After RC seconds, $V = V_0 \cdot e^{-1}$ and has thus fallen to about 37% of V_0; after the elapse of four time constants, more than 98% of the volume has been expired.

Average values for C of $0.15 \text{l} \cdot \text{cmH}_2\text{O}^{-1}$ ($1.5 \text{l} \cdot \text{kPa}^{-1}$) and for R of $2 \text{cmH}_2\text{O} \cdot \text{l}^{-1} \cdot \text{s}$ ($0.2 \text{kPa} \cdot \text{l}^{-1} \cdot \text{s}$) give a time constant of 0.3 s. Four time constants thus yield 1.2 s as an estimate of the adequate time for passive deflation of the lungs. Actual measurements of T_E in man at rest and for ventilations up to ca. $60 \text{l} \cdot \text{min}^{-1}$ are, however, considerably longer (Figure 1.3). This indicates that expiratory braking occurs.

Diaphragmatic and external intercostal muscle activity are known to continue into expiration, thereby pulling against the elastic forces acting at the onset of expiration and prolonging expiration. Recent studies (e.g. Shee *et al.*, 1985) have shown that while the pressure developed by the inspiratory muscles during expiration falls most steeply over the early part of expiration, it may continue for up to 80% of T_E. The post-inspiratory contraction of inspiratory muscles decreases at higher levels of drive and eventually ceases altogether.

Another factor responsible for the determination of the duration of an expiration of a given volume is clearly the **airway resistance**. Partitioning of total airway resistance tells us that about 90% can be attributed to the upper airways and bronchi greater than ca. 2 mm in diameter, of which again more than half is accounted for by the larynx. Increases in respiratory drive are associated with a fall in expiratory airway resistance. Both direct observations and EMG recordings have shown that the main laryngeal abductor, the posterior cricoarytaenoid muscle, is increasingly activated at greater respiratory drives when the demands for expiratory flow increase.

At much greater drives, on the other hand, the opposite occurs.

Once expiration becomes 'active' by contraction of the internal intercostal and the abdominal muscles in particular, then an additional rise of intrathoracic pressure will add to the elastic recoil forces and speed up expiration.

1.5 Neural influences

1.5.1 *Reflexes from the lungs*

Reference has already been made to the Hering-Breuer inflation reflex which is mediated by **slowly-adapting stretch receptors** innervated by myelinated fibres in the vagus nerve. However, it has long been known that the respiratory effects of vagotomy are different from the effects of merely abolishing the Hering-Breuer reflex, and also that inflation occasionally leads to positive feedback with an increased diaphragmatic activity and 'augmented' breaths. This response, known as Head's 'paradoxical reflex', was originally observed in rabbits after partial cooling of the vagus. Clearly, therefore, there are vagal receptors apart from stretch receptors that can affect breathing pattern. These are the rapidly-adapting receptors and those innervated by unmyelinated C fibres.

The **rapidly-adapting receptors**, previously called irritant receptors, are located in the airway mucosa and are probably particularly important for protective reflexes including mucus secretion. Coughing is the response to mechanical or chemical stimulation of those receptors located in the upper airways, while bronchoconstriction and hyperpnoea with a shortening of T_E are seen when more peripherally-located receptors are stimulated. These rapidly-adapting receptors are also thought to mediate the deflation reflex, and have recently been shown to respond to the rate of flow in the airways and, to a smaller extent, also to volume.

Since many stimuli are not unique or specific to one kind of receptor, attempts at distinguishing between effects caused by different vagal receptors have, of necessity, involved selective blocking procedures: both cooling of the vagus (to 8°C) and SO_2 inhalation (200 ppm) have been found to abolish the Hering-Breuer reflex. Davies *et al.* (1978) thus studied the breathing pattern of rabbits during air- and CO_2-breathing in the control state, during SO_2 inhalation with the Hering-Breuer reflex abolished, and after vagotomy. The effects of vagotomy clearly differed from those of selective stretch receptor inhibition, indicating that the rapidly-adapting receptors (and possibly also unmyelinated fibres) exert a shortening effect on both T_I and T_E.

Of the unmyelinated broncho-pulmonary **C-fibres**, the **J-receptors** (juxta-capillary) have been studied most intensively, notably by Paintal (1970). Injection of diphenylguanide in the right atrium stimulates the J-receptors after a short delay and leads to a reflex response which includes apnoea followed by rapid, shallow breathing with a shortened T_E.

1.5.2 *Pulmonary vagal receptors and CO_2*

The lungs of birds and lizards contain CO_2-sensitive receptors which inhibit the respiratory centres through vagal afferents. The discharge of these receptors is inversely related to the pulmonary PCO_2.

Breathing in mammals is also influenced by changes of airway PCO_2. In dogs on cardiopulmonary bypass, Bartoli *et al.* (1974) thus found that an increase of airway PCO_2 at a constant, unchanged arterial PCO_2 and PO_2 induced a rise of ventilation by a vagal reflex. This was predominantly caused by an increase of frequency due to a shortening of T_E with little change of T_I. It was claimed that this lung-CO_2 reflex was caused by a CO_2-induced depression of pulmonary stretch receptors, largely those which are still active at end-expiration (Bradley *et al.*, 1976). However, the involvement of other receptors could not be excluded, and later work by Coleridge *et al.* (1978) did establish that rapidly-adapting receptors also are activated by a fall and inhibited by a rise of airway PCO_2. Impulse activity in the unmyelinated C-fibres, on the other hand, was hardly affected.

The effect is due to a direct action of CO_2 on the receptor endings rather than to mechanical changes, and is most marked for values of PCO_2 less than about 20 mmHg (2.7 kPa). The effect is still present, but is much smaller, over the PCO_2 range 30–50 mmHg (4.0–6.7 kPa). It has therefore been claimed that the main functional significance of this reflex is to protect against the effects of a low PCO_2 associated with hyperventilation, and that its role in eucapnic breathing is trivial. However, it could be argued that during normal air-breathing the airways are exposed to a continuously changing PCO_2 in respired gas, decreasing toward zero during inspiration and rising rapidly to alveolar values during expiration. It is thus possible that the CO_2 sensitivity of the lung receptors may provide a phasic modulation of vagal feedback to the respiratory centres, but further work is clearly needed to establish whether this happens and, if so, its physiological significance.

1.5.3 *Afferent inputs*

This chapter has so far concentrated on breathing pattern in the steady state. We might provisionally interpret the quoted observations to imply that the ultimate output pattern of the respiratory centres is the same irrespective of the nature and source of the input (with the exception of temperature), be it predominantly mediated by the arterial chemoreceptors as in hypoxia, by central chemoreceptors as in hyperoxic hypercapnia, or be it of mixed origin as in exercise.

This interpretation implies an ultimate **convergence of inputs**, for which evidence has been presented in the cat by Loeschcke & Schlaefke (e.g. Loeschcke, 1982) and Millhorn *et al.* (1982). Thus, cooling of the 'intermediate' area on the ventrolateral surface of the medulla depresses and eventually suppresses responses to stimulation of the central chemosensitive areas and also, although not entirely, of the arterial chemoreceptors. Furthermore, Spode (e.g. Loeschcke, 1982) reported that stimulation of the ventral roots in the upper part of the lumbar cord had no respiratory effect when central chemosentivity was abolished by cooling. However, Millhorn *et al.* (1982) found the respiratory effects of electrical stimulation of muscle afferents to persist after cooling, indicating that at least some impulses from muscle may reach respiratory neurones without passing through the intermediate area. Also, the respiratory effects of thermal stimulation of the hypothalamus persist after cold block of the intermediate area.

1.6 **Dynamic changes of breathing pattern**

1.6.1 *Nature and time course of responses to different stimuli*

The respiratory centres may be considered a network of neurones to which sensory input gains access through many different pathways. So, although a final convergence of many of these inputs takes place, it is possible that the initial nature of the response and the time course of the changes might differ with different kinds of stimuli.

Such differences have indeed been reported for both cat and man. The findings reported by Gardner (1980) for humans will be briefly summarised:

(a) step changes of $P_{ET}O_2$ into hypoxia at a constant $P_{ET}CO_2$ affect frequency earlier than tidal volume, the earliest change being a marked shortening of T_E;
(b) step increases of $P_{ET}CO_2$ at a constant high $P_{ET}O_2$ (250 mmHg) cause an initial lengthening of T_I, which precedes changes in tidal volume.

In Figure 1.3, the initial T_E shortening in the hypoxic steps and T_I lengthening in the hypercapnic steps are indicated by the curved arrows; the steady-state V_T-T_E and V_T-T_I relationships (heavy lines) are only reached some 3 min after the onset of the step changes. The qualitative aspect of these responses has recently been confirmed by Robbins (1984) who used sinusoidal forcings of $P_{ET}O_2$ and/or $P_{ET}CO_2$.

Forcing methods used in dynamic studies include pulses, steps or sinusoidal changes in alveolar gas tensions. These produce rapid responses which can selectively affect an inspiratory or an expiratory component of the breathing pattern. Rebreathing from confined space may be considered equal to a ramp forcing or to a succession of small steps. The marked initial frequency effect (shortening of T_E) in the hypoxic steps is consistent with reports, dating back to Haldane, that breathing frequency during rebreathing tests changes rather more in relation to tidal volume when hypoxia is the predominant respiratory stimulus than when the central chemical drive dominates.

For exercise the dynamic pattern may differ according to the nature of the exercise and the magnitude of the step. Thus, in steps from rest to a moderate work rate, we have commonly found an initial rise of frequency due to a shortening of both inspiratory and expiratory durations preceding the rise of tidal volume. Between work rates, on the other hand, the changes of pattern tend to follow the steady state.

1.6.2 *The timing effect*

The timing effect is a feature or a property of the respiratory centres. This has been known for several years and has attracted much attention, in particular with respect to brainstem input from the arterial chemoreceptors (Black & Torrance, 1971). The respiratory response to a pulse or a step change differs according to the **timing of the stimulus in relation to the phase of the respiratory cycle**. An identical CO_2 pulse injected at the carotid body or an identical train of electrical stimuli of carotid sinus nerve afferents will thus have different effects if applied early or late during the inspiratory phase or during expiration.

The effects of regularly occurring breath-to-breath alternations of the time profile of alveolar PCO_2 at constant $P_{ET}CO_2$ on the pattern of breathing in man have been studied in our laboratory (Metias *et al.*, 1981; Cunningham *et al.*, 1986). Changes between two inspiratory gas mixtures, one with a high PCO_2 and one with a low, were triggered during inspiration such that, on one breath, the early part of an inspiration had a high PCO_2 and the late part a low PCO_2, while on the next breath the order was reversed (low PCO_2 early, high PCO_2 late), and so on. Only when imposed on a constant hypoxic background ($P_{ET}O_2$ ca. 55mmHg or 7.3kPa) did these PCO_2 changes regularly produce breath-to-breath alternations of one or more of the respiratory output variables. This, along with the observed latencies, indicates an **arterial chemoreceptor** origin. Alternation of inspiratory variables in the absence of expiratory alternation was commonly seen.

These studies provide evidence for discrete accessibility of information carried by the **carotid sinus nerve** to neurones in the brainstem influencing mainly or exclusively inspiratory or expiratory flows, volumes or durations, the exact nature of the response being dependent on the timing. Furthermore, the high incidence of regular alternation of either inspiratory or expiratory variables indicates that the effects are short lasting – 'forgotten' already in the next breath.

The timing effect is potentially of very considerable interest, and there is now substantial evidence that the transducive properties of the arterial chemoreceptors allow coding and signalling of the information contained in the oscillations of arterial PO_2, PCO_2 and pH (see chapter 4 for detailed discussion).

In the steady-state of exercise, the timing of arrival at the brainstem of some peak or trough activity related to an oscillating impulse activity in the carotid sinus nerve would be expected to be fixed to a certain part of the central phase of either inspiration or expiration, provided breathing is regular. We do, however, know that regular breathing is frequently interrupted because of swallowing, sighing, etc. Following such interruptions, a shift in the phase relationship between chemoreceptor impulses and central respiratory rhythmicity would be expected to occur, and this in turn might affect the respiratory response (Cunningham, 1975).

We therefore investigated whether any reflex effects on ventilation during exercise could be related to spontaneous phase shifts (Petersen *et al.*, 1978). We were unable to demonstrate any such effects, and so – although much evidence favours the significance of the timing effect – it appears to be too small during euoxic exercise in man to be detected by the means available (see chapter 5 for detailed discussion).

1.6.3 *The duration of inspiration*

It has been suggested that negative feedback from the pulmonary stretch receptors contributes importantly to the control of inspiratory duration, although its importance during eupnoeic breathing in man may be queried. Non-vagal factors that may influence inspiratory time include impulses originating in the nucleus parabrachialis medialis (NPBM) in the upper pons (also termed the **pneumotaxic centre**). Cohen (1979) and others have reported, for example, that discrete stimuli in this region induce a premature termination of inspiration. Also, impulses originating in the chest wall – excited by compression of the chest or by vibration – may influence T_I probably through stimulation of intercostal muscle spindles. And reference has already been made to the tonic influence of a raised body temperature, which acts to shorten both T_I and T_E.

The inspiratory 'off-switch' model proposed by von Euler (1983) is compatible with many experimental findings and has provoked much interest and work in this area. The model suggests that an **inspiratory-terminating off-switch mechanism** is activated when a rising **centrally-generated inspiratory activity** (CIA), in combination with the increasing afferent pulmonary stretch receptor activity, reaches a certain threshold value. Once this has happened, the upper bulbo-spinal inspiratory motorneurones are inhibited and remain so for the subsequent expiration. Following vagotomy, CIA must rise to a higher level before the off-switch threshold is reached, and inspiration is therefore prolonged. Were the off-switch threshold also to be raised, a further prolongation of inspiration would be expected to occur. An example of this, which has been known for a long time, is apneustic breathing characterised by prolonged inspiratory efforts interrupted by brief expirations. Apneusis may be induced in experimental animals by the combination of vagotomy with either a mid-pontine transection of the brainstem or with discrete lesions in the NPBM. According to the Euler model, structures in the NPBM normally exert a threshold-lowering influence on the inspiratory off-switch mechanism.

The specificity of the NPBM with regard to the pneumotaxic centre has, however, been queried. For example, St. John (1972) observed apneusis in anaesthetised cats with chronic NPBM lesions and bilateral vagotomy but, following withdrawal of the anaesthesia, apneusis was converted into eupnoea. It was concluded that other areas of the central nervous system can compensate for the pontine pneumotaxic effects.

The shortening of inspiration seen in response to a raised body temperature may be explained as an off-switch threshold-lowering effect, possibly mediated by descending hypothalamic projections.

Euler's inspiratory off-switch mechanism was originally considered an all-or-none phenomenon. Later work by Younes *et al.* (1978) has, however, established that it is a progressive, graded event, which is reversible for part of its course.

1.6.4 *The duration of expiration*

The principal factors governing expiratory flow have already been discussed. At low respiratory drives, changes in both upper airway (mainly laryngeal) resistance and in post-inspiratory muscle contraction contribute to expiratory braking. At greater respiratory drives, the high expiratory flows encountered are caused by active expiratory efforts through the abdominal muscles.

These expiratory flow-controlling mechanisms are governed by chemical stimuli as well as by mechanical feedback from the vagus.

Once the chemical drive to breathing has set or planned the time course of expiratory flow, continuous monitoring of flow and volume (presumably by rapidly-adapting receptors, as well as by pulmonary stretch receptors) will allow corrections for deviations from the planned time course by appropriate compensatory reflex adjustments.

Remmers & Bartlett (1977) studied unanaesthetised cats with chronic tracheostomies which could be opened or closed by remote control. Closing the tracheostomy during expiration (and thereby increasing the upper airway resistance) caused a decrease of diaphragmatic activity and increased activity of the posterior cricoarytaenoid muscle (i.e., a widening of the glottis) and the abdominal muscles. These changes, which compensated for the increased airway resistance, continued throughout expiration. Following opening of the tracheostomy, the opposite changes were observed. While these findings may have provided a reasonable understanding of the regulation and continuous 'tracking' of expiratory flow, far less is still known about the mechanisms that actually terminate expiration or 'trigger' the following inspiration. Remmers & Bartlett found that the flow changes caused by opening and closing the tracheostomy were accompanied by changes of expiratory time: a decreased expiratory airflow, whether caused by closing the tracheostomy (in turn increasing the airway resistance) or by opening the tracheostomy (and thus increasing diaphragmatic and laryngeal braking) was accompanied by an increased T_E. The timing of the triggering of the next inspiration was thus related to the expiratory flow pattern, but was independent of the nature of the 'tracking' response. Both responses were eliminated by vagotomy.

Attempts at answering the question about the initiation of inspiration have operated with the concept of a **central expiratory-controlling activity** which inhibits expiratory-inspiratory switching. This activity declines with time and will eventually allow inspiration to start. The findings of Remmers & Bartlett (1977) may add a **peripheral volume-related inhibition** to this scheme. As lung volume, and thence the inhibition, decreases with time during expiration, the total inhibition of the mechanism responsible for the expiratory-inspiratory transition may thus have two components: one set by the central drive, and one by volume-related feedback. This basic concept is supported by work by Cohen (1979), who found that application of brief tetanic stimuli to a discrete area of the rostral pons during expiration could initiate inspiration. The minimal stimulus intensity required to bring about this effect was found to decrease with time during expiration.

Based upon studies of brainstem respiratory neurones, Richter (1982) has recently suggested that expiration should be subdivided into two stages. Stage 1 is characterised by a declining phrenic activity, while stage 2 is silent or – if the respiratory drive is sufficiently strong – is characterised by active expiratory motor activity. The inspiratory activity in stage 1 is considered to represent a separate activity, not merely a slow decline of phrenic discharge following the termination of inspiration.

1.7 **The neural drive**

It is possible to assess the output of the respiratory centres – the **neural drive** – by recording the phrenic electroneurogram (ENG) or the diaphragmatic EMG. In healthy man both ventilation and mean inspiratory flow are regarded as acceptable indices of the total drive. However, although ventilation ($\dot{V}$) and mean inspiratory flow (V_T/T_I) appear to be linearly related over a wide range of drives, they do not change proportionately. This is implicit in the breathing pattern responses to changing drive shown in Figure 1.3 (T_E changes more than T_I). The same conclusion may be reached by a simple algebraic treatment of eqn (1.1) (Milic-Emili *et al.*, 1975). Thus, rearranging,

$$\dot{V} = V_T \cdot f = V_T \cdot (1/T_{tot}) = (V_T/T_I) \cdot (T_I/T_{tot}) \qquad (1.3)$$

in which V_T/T_I may be considered a drive-related index and T_I/T_{tot} a timing index, which is also referred to as the **inspiratory duty cycle**.

Since $T_I/T_{tot} = 1/(1 + T_E/T_I)$, any disproportionate change of T_I and T_E will affect the relationship between $\dot{V}$ and V_T/T_I. When ventilation increases in man, both V_T/T_I and T_I/T_{tot} typically increase. The rise of T_I/T_{tot} reflects simply that T_I in range 1 changes considerably less than T_E. The basic advantage of this approach over the simpler $\dot{V} = V_T \times f$ is that the volume-time relationship during inspiration in man is usually linear, which means that V_T/T_I is independent of T_I, while V_T is determined by both inspiratory flow and T_I.

The efficiency of diaphragmatic and intercostal contractions in generating pressure as well as the conversion of pressure changes into air flow are, however, subject to various influences. The pressure generated by muscular contraction is related to the length and geometry of the muscle. With an increased lung volume, both external intercostal and diaphragmatic fibres become shorter and hence develop less force on stimulation. The flattening of the diaphragm at large lung volumes also decreases the development of pressure. The associated pressure-volume and pressure-flow relationships are determined by mechanical factors, basically the compliance and the airway resistance, and differ between individuals.

A more satisfactory index of the neural drive to breathing is probably the **mouth occlusion pressure** (Whitelaw *et al.*, 1975). The measurement of this involves recording of the pressure in the mouth during inspiration against an occluded airway, from which two indices may be derived: the pressure at 0.1 s ($P_{0.1}$) or the maximum rate of rise of pressure during the occluded inspiration. Because of the pressure-length considerations mentioned above, measurements must be made at the lungs' equilibrium volume (FRC).

Occlusion pressure may be considered a parallel to the use of dP/dt max during the isovolumetric part of ventricular systole as an inotropic index. In studies on both cat and man, it has been found to be linearly related to the integrated diaphragmatic EMG and to the phrenic ENG.

1.8 The work and O_2 cost of breathing

The metabolic cost involved in the mechanical work of breathing in healthy individuals is very small during eupnoea, hardly exceeding more than a few percent of the resting metabolic rate.

At higher ventilations, both the elastic and flow-resistive work of breathing increase, and the O_2 cost of breathing thus rises steeply. Measurements are difficult, but values of 15–20% of the total O_2 uptake have been reported for ventilations above

$100 l \cdot min^{-1}$. Such values have been indirectly confirmed by measurements of diaphragmatic blood flow and arterio-venous O_2 differences in the dog (e.g. Bye *et al.*, 1983). In patients with obstructive lung disease, much higher values have been found (up to 40% of the O_2 uptake at low ventilations).

Ventilatory increments in exercise are therefore associated with an energy sharing between respiratory and non-respiratory muscles, in which a progressively larger and larger fraction is required by the respiratory muscles. Eventually the total energy requirements may exceed the supply, and either or both of the two muscle groups may suffer from an inadequate O_2 supply causing anaerobiosis and decreased force development.

At low ventilations, neither the force which has to be developed by the respiratory muscles nor the mechanical work of breathing is likely to be influenced significantly by changes in breathing pattern. Earlier analyses and suggestions by Otis *et al.* (1950) and Mead (1960) have been followed up by the application of modern control theory in the study of optimisation: whether the respiratory system selects a pattern of breathing which minimises respiratory work (Grodins & Yamashiro, 1979). However, while such theoretical studies have indeed indicated that optimisation may become increasingly important at higher ventilations, they cannot establish the nature of the physiological mechanisms responsible for the selection of an optimum pattern, and there is so far no satisfactory answer to this question.

The ideas of optimisation are compatible with the general observation (see above) of a unique steady-state pattern in man, which is related to the total ventilation, irrespective of the nature of the drive and the metabolic rate.

1.9 **A note about measurement**

Human subjects have conventionally been studied while breathing through a mouthpiece with a noseclip or through a face mask. It has often been claimed that these means of measurement by themselves affect breathing, generally toward a deeper and slower pattern. There is, however, still no general agreement, either about the precise qualitative nature of the induced changes or about the mechanisms involved.

Observed changes in breathing pattern may not be induced by the measuring devices themselves, but may be an indirect consequence of a shift from nose to mouth breathing. Such a shift would by itself imply a decrease in upper airway resistance that might affect the pressure-flow relationship. It has also been suggested that receptors in the mouth and pharynx are affected by changes in the temperature of the inspired air, as occurs with a shift from nose to mouth breathing. But it is still possible that observed changes are entirely unspecific cortical responses.

Any effects related to the method of measurement, whatever their cause, are most likely to affect ventilation at rest and at low drives. It is well known that rest is a particularly difficult condition to study. The 'noise' level may be very high, and hyperventilation is common in subjects unfamiliar with respiratory testing. If the route of entry of inspired air is important, then – on the assumption that unimpeded breathing changes from predominantly nose-breathing to predominantly mouth-breathing at ventilations of ca. $25–30 \, \mathrm{l \cdot min^{-1}}$ – it is unlikely that mouthpiece-noseclip breathing should have any significant effects at higher intensities of drive.

The method of respiratory inductive plethysmography ('Respitrace') was introduced a few years ago in an attempt to provide a non-invasive method of recording of respiratory movements (Sackner *et al.*, 1980). The device consists of coils of teflon-insulated wire sewn into elastic bands, which are positioned about the rib cage and abdomen. Changes in the self-inductance of the coils caused by volume changes provide a signal which, with appropriate calibration, reflects V_T. The method permits separation of the abdominal and costal contributions to breathing and has proved useful in several situations. It is particularly well suited for studies of breathing at rest, during sleep and for routine studies in patients.

1.10 **Concluding comments**

The respiratory system is characterised by a remarkable flexibility which enables it both to adapt to changing demands for O_2 and CO_2 transport and to adjust and correct for transient disturbances. The emphasis of this chapter has been on the pattern of breathing, i.e. the way in which a given ventilatory response is brought about.

The dynamics of the system have been studied by different forcing methods: pulses, steps or sinusoidal changes in alveolar gas tensions or work rate. The responses to such forcings are rapid, often selectively affecting either an inspiratory or an expiratory component with very little after-effect. This indicates a short-memory control, the precise nature of which may differ according to the source and timing of the triggering input.

Some inputs may both arise and induce corrective changes of respiration within the course of a single breath. This applies to impulses from muscle or from vagal afferents from the lungs. Other inputs provide a reflex response which is delayed in relation to the event that initiated it. For the carotid body, for example, the delay caused by the circulatory transit time from the lungs is usually in the order of two breaths.

The establishment of a steady state takes minutes to develop and is characterised by a remarkably similar pattern, irrespective of the nature and source of the driving stimulus. In the steady state, a given rise of ventilation induced by the inhalation of an hypoxic or a hypercapnic gas mixture or by exercise is achieved by basically the same changes of T_I, T_E and V_T. This indicates the presence of control mechanisms concerned with the management of *total* ventilation as distinct from the overall control of ventilation in relation to the demands for gas exchange set by the rate of tissue metabolism. Since the work of breathing in a given individual is related to ventilation, this then would appear to be the kind of control which should be expected to occur at some stage in the central breath generation for optimisation to take place.

This chapter has only touched upon the central nervous mechanisms subserving respiratory regulation and control. By repeated reference to work done on the intact, unanaesthetised human subject, it has however attempted to define some operational properties of the respiratory centres related to speed of adjustments, to flexibility and capacity for change, and to economy of performance. One additional important feature of respiratory control is its homeostatic nature. Over a wide range of metabolic rates, ventilation is so finely adjusted to gas-exchange rates that PCO_2 and pH in arterial blood and extracellular fluids including that of the brain are maintained within narrow limits. This homeostatic control is discussed in the other chapters in this book.

1.11 Further reading

Hornbein, T. F., ed. (1981). *Regulation of Breathing*. Chapters by: J. G. Widdicombe, Nervous receptors in the respiratory tract and lungs; R. A. Mitchell & A. J. Berger. Neural regulation of respiration; M. K. Younes & J. E. Remmers, Control of tidal volume and respiratory frequency: J. Milic-Emili, W. A. Whitelaw & A. E. Grassino. Measurement and testing of respiratory drive; F. S. Grodins, Models. Dekker, New York.

References

Bartoli, A., Cross, B. A., Guz, A., Jain, S. K., Noble, M. I. M. & Trenchard, D. (1974). The effect of carbon dioxide in the airways and alveoli on ventilation; a vagal reflex studied in the dog. *Journal of Physiology*, **240**, 91–109.

Black, A. M. S. & Torrance, R. W. (1971). Respiratory oscillations in chemoreceptor discharge in the control of breathing. *Respiration Physiology*, **13**, 221–37.

Bradley, G. W., Noble, M. I. M. & Trenchard, D. (1976). The direct effect of pulmonary stretch receptor discharge produced by changing lung carbon dioxide concentration in dogs on cardiopulmonary bypass and its action on breathing. *Journal of Physiology*, **261**, 359–73.

Brody, A. W. (1954). Mechanical compliance and resistance of the lung-thorax calculated from the flow recorded during passive expiration. *American Journal of Physiology*, **178**, 189–96.

Bye, P. T. P., Farkas, G. A. & Roussos, Ch. (1983). Respiratory factors limiting exercise. *Annual Review of Physiology*, **45**, 439–51.

Cohen, M. I. (1979). Neurogenesis of respiratory rhythm in the mammal. *Physiological Reviews*, **59**, 1105–73.

Coleridge, H. M., Coleridge, J. C.G. & Banzett, R. B. (1978). Effect of CO_2 on afferent vagal endings in the canine lung. *Respiration Physiology*, **24**, 135–51.

Cunningham, D. J. C. (1975). A model illustrating the importance of timing in the regulation of breathing. *Nature*, **253**, 440–42.

Cunningham, D. J. C., Howson, M. G., Metias, E. F. & Petersen, E. S. (1986). Patterns of breathing in response to alternating patterns of alveolar carbon dioxide pressures in man. *Journal of Physiology*, **376**, 31–45.

Davies, A., Dixon, M., Callanan, D., Huszcuk, A., Widdicombe, J. G. & Wise, J. C. M. (1978). Lung reflexes in rabbits during pulmonary stretch receptor block by sulphur dioxide. *Respiration Physiology*, **34**, 83–101.

Euler, C. von (1983). On the central pattern generator for the basic breathing rhythmicity. *Journal of Applied Physiology*, **55**, 1647–59.

Fry, D.L. & Hyatt, R.E. (1960). Pulmonary mechanics. A unified analysis of the relationship between pressure, volume, and gas flow in the lungs of normal and diseased human subjects. *American Journal of Medicine*, **29**, 672–89.

Gardner, W.N. (1977). The relation between tidal volume and inspiratory and expiratory times during steady-state carbon dioxide inhalation in man. *Journal of Physiology*, **272**, 591–611.

Gardner, W.N. (1980). The pattern of breathing following step changes of alveolar partial pressures of carbon dioxide and oxygen in man. *Journal of Physiology*, **300**, 55–73.

Garrard, C.S. & Lane, D.J. (1978). The pattern of stimulated breathing in man during non-elastic expiratory loading. *Journal of Physiology*, **279**, 17–29.

Grodins, F.S. & Yamashiro, S.M. (1979). What is the pattern of breathing regulated for? In: *Central Nervous Control Mechanisms in Breathing* (Euler, C. von & Lagercrantz, H., eds.), pp. 169–75. Pergamon, Oxford.

Guz, A., Noble, M.I.M., Eisele, J.H. & Trenchard, D. (1970). The role of vagal inflation reflexes in man and other animals. In: *Breathing: Hering-Breuer Centenary Symposium* (Porter, R., ed. pp. 17–40. Churchill, London.

Hyatt, R.E. (1983). Expiratory flow limitation. *Journal of Applied Physiology*, **55**, 1–8.

Jensen, J.I., Lyager, S. & Pedersen, O.F. (1980). The relationship between maximal ventilation, breathing pattern and mechanical limitation of ventilation. *Journal of Physiology*, **309**, 521–32.

Kay, J.D.S., Petersen, E.S. & Vejby-Christensen, H. (1975). Mean and breath-by-breath pattern of breathing in man during steady-state exercise. *Journal of Physiology*, **251**, 657–69.

Loeschcke, H.H. (1982). Central chemosensitivity and the reaction theory. *Journal of Physiology*, **332**, 1–24.

Mead, J. (1960). Control of respiratory frequency. *Journal of Applied Physiology*, **15**, 325–36.

Metias, E.F., Cunningham, D.J.C., Howson, M.G., Petersen, E.S. & Wolff, C.B. (1981). Reflex effects on human breathing of breath-by-breath changes of the time profile of alveolar PCO_2 during steady hypoxia. *Pflugers Archiv*, **389**, 243–50.

Milic-Emili, J., Mazzarelli, M., Derenne, J.-Ph., Whitelaw, W.A. & Couture, J. (1975). A new approach to study control of breathing. *Clinical Research*, **23**, 646A.

Millhorn, D.E., Eldridge, F.L. & Waldrop, T.G. (1982). Effects of medullary area I(s) cooling on respiratory response to muscle stimulation. *Respiration Physiology*, **49**, 41–48.

Newsom Davis, J. & Stagg, D. (1975). Interrelationships of the volume and time components of individual breaths in resting man. *Journal of Physiology*, **245**, 481–98.

Otis, A. B., Fenn, W. O. & Rahn, H. (1950). Mechanics of breathing in man. *Journal of Applied Physiology*, **2**, 592–607.

Paintal, A. S. (1970). The mechanism of excitation of type J receptors, and the J reflex. In: *Breathing: Hering-Breuer Centenary Symposium* (Porter, R., ed.) pp. 59–71. Churchill, London.

Petersen, E. S. & Vejby-Christensen, H. (1977). Effects of body temperature on ventilatory response to hypoxia and breathing pattern in man. *Journal of Applied Physiology*, **42**, 492–500.

Petersen, E. S., Whipp, B. J., Drysdale, D. B. & Cunningham, D. J. C. (1978). Carotid arterial blood gas oscillations and the phase of the respiratory cycle during exercise in man. Testing a model. In: *The Regulation of Respiration during Sleep and Anaesthesia* (Fitzgerald, R. S., Gautier, H. & Lahiri, S., eds.) pp. 335–42. Plenum Press, New York.

Priban, I. P. (1963). An analysis of some short-term patterns of breathing in man at rest. *Journal of Physiology*, **166**, 425–34.

Remmers, J. E. & Bartlett, D., Jr (1977). Reflex control of expiratory airflow and duration. *Journal of Applied Physiology*, **42**, 80–87.

Richter, D. W. (1982). Generation and maintenance of the respiratory rhythm. *Journal of Experimental Biology*, **100**, 93–107.

Robbins, P. A. (1984). The ventilatory response of the human respiratory system to sine waves of alveolar carbon dioxide and hypoxia. *Journal of Physiology*, **350**, 461–74.

Sackner, J. D., Nixon, A. J., Davis, B., Atkins, N. & Sackner, M. A. (1980). Non-invasive measurement of ventilation during exercise using a respiratory inductive plethysmograph. *American Review of Respiratory Disease*, **122**, 867–71.

Shee, C. D., Ploy-Song-Sang, Y. & Milic-Emili, J. (1985). Decay of inspiratory muscle pressure during exercise in conscious humans. *Journal of Applied Physiology*, **58**, 1859–65.

St. John, W. M. (1972). Respiratory tidal volume responses of cats with chronic pneumotaxic center lesions. *Respiration Physiology*, **16**, 92–108.

Whitelaw, W. A., Derenne, J.-Ph. & Milic-Emili, J. (1975). Occlusion pressure as a measure of respiratory centre output in conscious man. *Respiration Physiology*, **23**, 181–99.

Younes, M., Remmers, J. E. & Baker, J. (1978). Characteristics of inspiratory inhibition by phasic volume feedback in cats. *Journal of Applied Physiology*, **40**, 177–83.

2

The ventilatory response to hypoxia

S. A. Ward and P. A. Robbins Department of Anesthesiology, University of California, Los Angeles and University Laboratory of Physiology, Oxford University

2.1 **Introduction**

Arterial hypoxaemia is encountered in conditions which are associated with a reduction in the ambient PO_2 as at altitude, and/or disease induced impairments of pulmonary gas exchange. Moderate degrees of hypoxaemia do not result in striking increases in ventilation ($\dot{V}_E$); however, when additional drives such as hypercapnia and exercise are imposed concurrently, a marked $\dot{V}_E$ response may occur. Controlled manipulations of this kind have provided much information about the operation of the ventilatory control system, and it is with such responses that this chapter is primarily concerned.

2.2 **Steady-state characteristics**

The steady-state relationship between $\dot{V}_E$ and alveolar[1] (end-tidal) PO_2 ($P_{ET}O_2$) is curvilinear (Figure 2.1). In eucapnia, the relationship is flat over the normal range of $P_{ET}O_2$ with little discernible stimulation occurring until $P_{ET}O_2$ falls to about 60 mmHg (8.0 kPa). Further reductions in $P_{ET}O_2$ however, increase the slope progressively. It is important to recognise that if care is not taken to prevent the resultant fall of arterial PCO_2

[1]Although alveolar PO_2 is widely used in such formulations, it should be recognized that the hypoxic stimulus to $\dot{V}_E$ derives from arterial PO_2 (as sensed by the carotid chemoreceptors). This is an important distinction in conditions, such as pulmonary disease, where the alveolar-to-arterial PO_2 difference is widened.

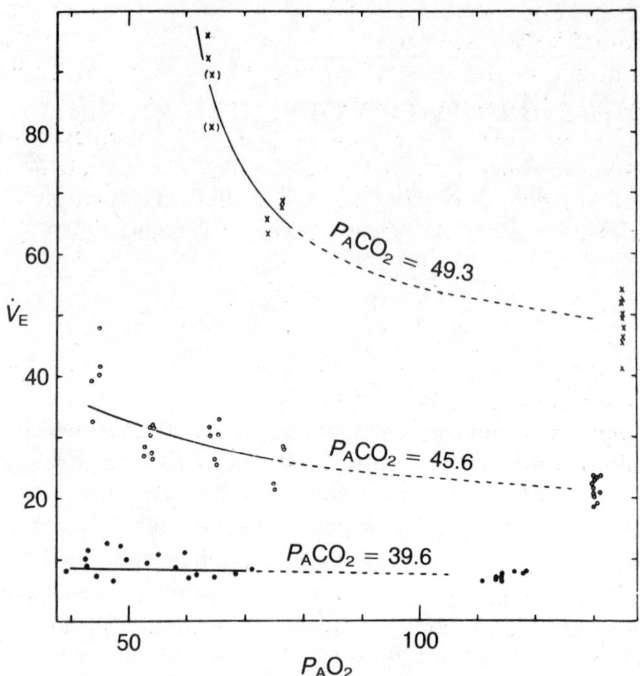

Fig. 2.1 Steady-state relationships between ventilation ($\dot{V}_E$) and alveolar PO_2 (P_AO_2) at three levels of alveolar PCO_2 (P_ACO_2). (From Lloyd & Cunningham, 1963.)

(P_aCO_2), the constraining influence of the hypocapnia will result in underestimation of the primary $\dot{V}_E$ response to the hypoxia.

A hyperbolic function has been traditionally used to describe the isocapnic $\dot{V}_E$-$P_{ET}O_2$ relationship. For example, Lloyd & Cunningham (1963) have defined **hypoxic sensitivity** (A) in terms of the *proportional* increase in $\dot{V}_E$ induced by hypoxia (i.e. relative to the hyperoxic value of $\dot{V}_E$)

$$\dot{V}_E = \dot{V}_E\,(0) + \dot{V}_E\,(0) \cdot A/(P_{ET}O_2 - C)$$

or,

$$\dot{V}_E/\dot{V}_E\,(0) = 1 + A/(P_{ET}O_2 - C) \qquad (2.1)$$

where $\dot{V}_E$ is the response at a particular $P_{ET}O_2$; $\dot{V}_E(0)$ is the response during hyperoxia which, in man, is assumed to 'silence' the carotid bodies (see below); C is an asymptotic level of $P_{ET}O_2$ (averaging 32 mmHg or 4.3 kPa); and A is the hypoxic sensitivity (averaging 23 mmHg or 3.1 kPa in eucapnia).

Weil *et al.* (1970) have used a slightly different expression, however, in which the hypoxic sensitivity (A') is related to the *absolute* increase of $\dot{V}_E$ induced by hypoxia (and averages 127 mmHg · 1 · min^{-1} or 953 kPa · 1 · min^{-1} (in eucapnia)

$$\dot{V}_E = \dot{V}_E\,(0) + A'/(P_{ET}O_2 - C) \qquad (2.2)$$

These formulations are discussed in greater detail by Cunningham (1974) and Rebuck & Slutsky (1981).

Exponential characterisations of the $\dot{V}_E$-$P_{ET}O_2$ relationship have also been proposed, such as that of Kronenberg *et al.* (1972)

$$\dot{V}_E - \dot{V}_E\,(0) = [\dot{V}_E\,(\infty) - \dot{V}_E\,(0)] \cdot e^{-P_{ET}O_2/K} \qquad (2.3)$$

where $\dot{V}_E\,(\infty)$ is the response to an infinitely large hypoxic stimulus; and the exponent, K, is the **hypoxic constant** (averaging 24.5 mmHg or 3.3 kPa in eucapnia).

Cherniack *et al.* (1971) and Rebuck & Campbell (1974) demonstrated that the $\dot{V}_E$-$P_{ET}O_2$ relationship can be linearised by expressing $\dot{V}_E$ as a function of arterial O_2 saturation (S_aO_2)

$$\dot{V}_E = G \cdot S_aO_2 + \dot{V}_E(0) \qquad (2.4)$$

where the slope G is the **hypoxic sensitivity** (averaging 1.47 l · min^{-1} · %$^{-1}$ in eucapnia). This is because the relationship between S_aO_2 and P_aO_2 can be shown to be well described by an exponential function over the S_aO_2 range of 35% to 100% (Severinghaus, 1976)

$$100 - S_aO_2 = 1.89^{-0.05 P_aO_2} \qquad (2.5)$$

Assuming alveolar and arterial PO_2 to be similar, the linearity of the $\dot{V}_E$-S_aO_2 relationship is thus compatible with an exponential

$\dot{V}_E$-P_aO_2 relationship. The utility of S_aO_2 lies in the ease with which it can be monitored continuously and non-invasively by ear oximetry (reviewed by Saunders *et al.*, 1976). However, characterisation of the hypoxic stimulus to $\dot{V}_E$ in terms of S_aO_2 rather than $P_{ET}O_2$ or P_aO_2 should not be taken to imply that the carotid chemoreceptors respond to SO_2 rather than PO_2; it is merely an empirical expedient.

Both the hyperbolic and exponential $\dot{V}_E$-$P_{ET}O_2$ formulations have been shown to provide adequate fits to the data over a range of approximately 40 to 120 mmHg (5.3 to 16.0 kPa), although the hyperbolic form has been more widely employed (see Cunningham, 1974, and Cunningham *et al.*, 1986, for detailed discussion). However, there appear to be no strong physiological grounds for distinguishing between these two descriptions over this range.

2.3 **Contribution of the carotid bodies to hypoxic sensitivity**

These organs have been shown to be the most important transducer of hypoxia for the human ventilatory control system. Evidence supporting this contention derives from several sources.

(a) Local anaesthetic blockade of the IXth and Xth cranial nerves (and presumably traffic from the carotid and aortic bodies) abolished the $\dot{V}_E$ response to hypoxia (Guz *et al.*, 1966).
(b) $\dot{V}_E$ does not increase with hypoxia in subjects whose carotid bodies have been denervated (either unintentionally during carotid endarterectomy surgery or by carotid body resection) (reviewed by Whipp *et al.*, 1983) (Figure 2.2). However, a weak $\dot{V}_E$ response may occur in such subjects when caused to be simultaneously hypercapnic (Swanson *et al.*, 1978; Honda *et al.*, 1979) (Figure 2.2); this may involve the aortic bodies, the glomus pulmonale or regenerated carotid afferents.

There is also evidence to suggest that the carotid bodies in man are reversibly 'silenced' by hyperoxia (though not necessaily in other species). The latency of the fall in $\dot{V}_E$ resulting from abrupt, transient replacement of a hyperoxic-hypercapnic inspirate with hyperoxia was consistent with a central chemoreceptor response, rather than the shorter latency of a carotid body response (Miller *et al.*, 1974) (Figure 2.3); this suggests that the carotid chemoreceptors were inactive and thus unable to respond to the PCO_2 change. Ward & Bellville (1983) reached a similar conclusion based on the $\dot{V}_E$ response latency to a step-increase of end-tidal PCO_2 ($P_{ET}CO_2$) in euoxia at rest and during exercise.

2.4 Contribution of other mechanisms to hypoxic sensitivity

While the carotid bodies appear to be the primary mediators of the $\dot{V}_E$ response to hypoxia, other factors can assume importance when at the extremes of hypoxia and hyperoxia and may also contribute to the response obtained in the normal range. If account is not taken of these, spurious estimates of the actual carotid body sensitivity to hypoxia may result.

Marked Hyperoxia ($P_aO_2 > 400$ mmHg or 53.3 kPa).
When O_2 is breathed for a sustained period, $\dot{V}_E$ is found to be slightly greater than with air-breathing. This may reflect:

(a) a hyperoxic-induced cerebral hypoperfusion (Kety & Schmidt, 1948; Lambertsen *et al.*, 1953) leading to a rise of cerebral PCO_2 and a fall of pH and, in turn, stimulation of the central chemoreceptors;
(b) a smaller degree of haemoglobin desaturation in the cerebral vasculature owing to the extra O_2 physically dissolved in blood, so reducing the magnitude of the Haldane effect (Dautrebande & Haldane, 1922; Lambertsen *et al.*, 1953) such that, again, cerebral PCO_2 rises and pH falls.

Marked Hypoxia ($P_aO_2 < 50$ mmHg or 6.7 kPa).
Extreme hypoxia has been reported to evoke a cerebral metabolic acidosis via stimulation of anaerobic glycolysis (Ponten & Siesjo, 1966); the consequent fall of cerebral pH serving to increase $\dot{V}_E$. Hypoxia has also been shown to exert a depressant effect on $\dot{V}_E$ (Figure 2.4); although there is no consensus as to the critical P_aO_2 at which this effect becomes manifest in man (see Lahiri & Gelfand, 1981 and Whipp *et al.*, 1983). Two possible mechanisms may be involved:

(a) direct hypoxic depression of neuronal activity; and

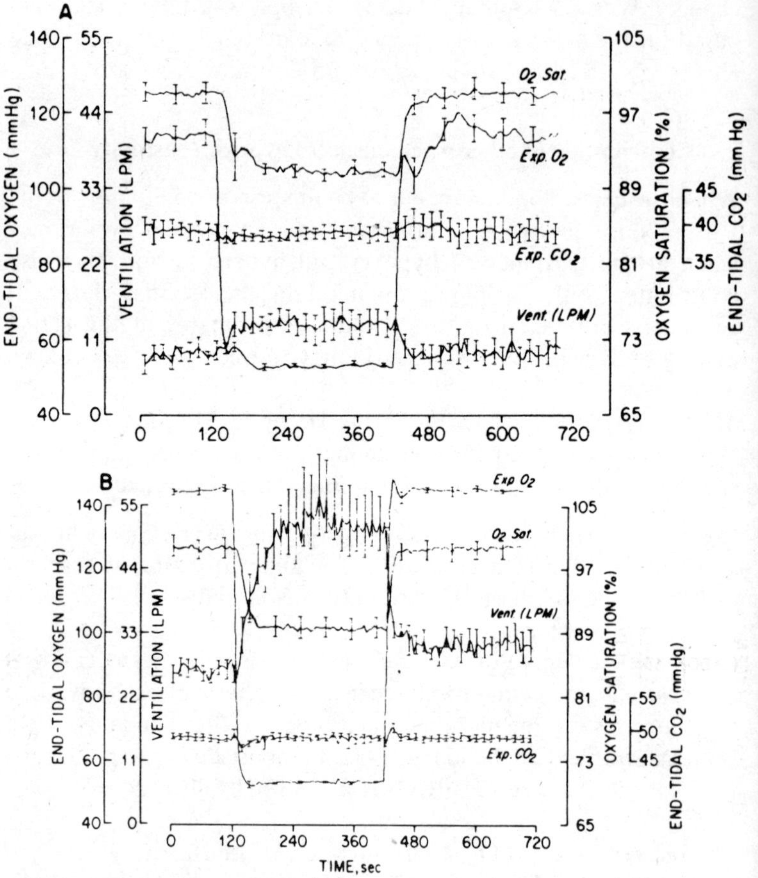

(*a*) A group of normal subjects.

Fig. 2.2 Ventilatory response ($1 \cdot min^{-1}$) to an isocapnic step-decrease in end-tidal PO_2. A: in eucapnia ($P_{ET}CO_2$ = 39 mmHg or 5.2 kPa). B: in hypercapnia ($P_{ET}CO_2$ = 49 mmHg or 6.5 kPa).

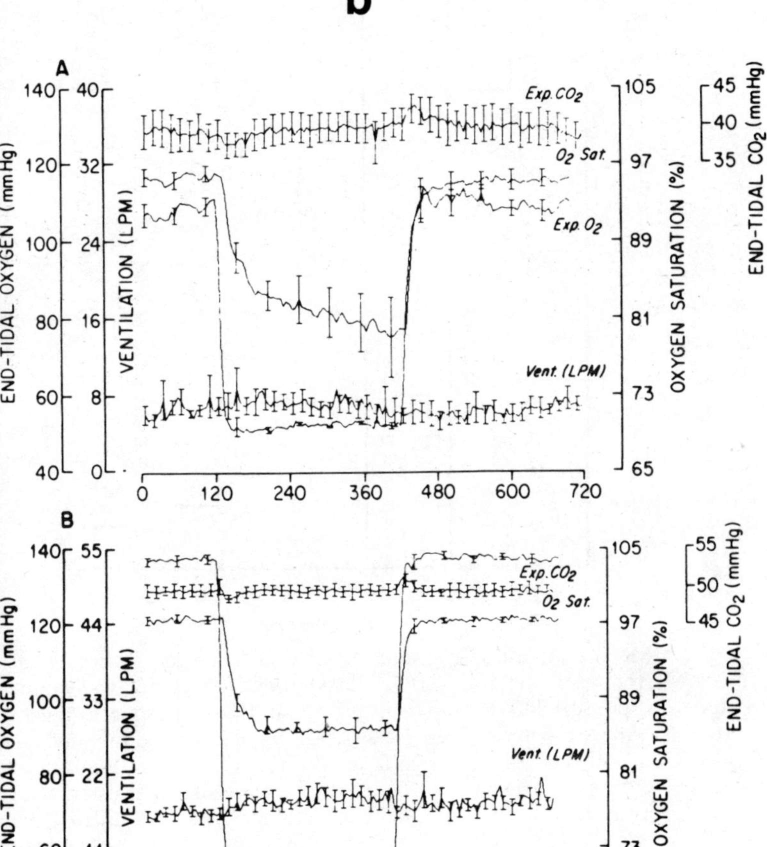

(*b*) A group of subjects who had previously undergone carotid body resection.

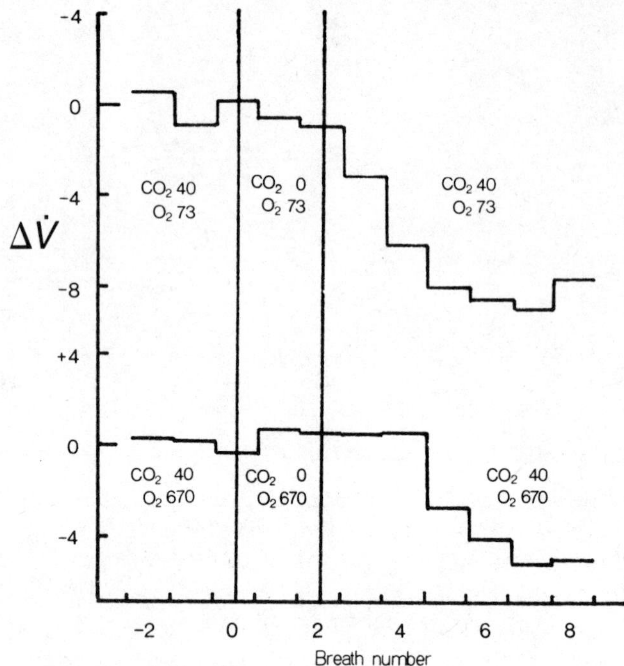

Fig. 2.3 Mean temporal response of ventilation ($\Delta\dot{V}$) to two breaths of pure O_2 (between the two vertical lines) against hypoxic-hypercapnic (upper response) and hyperoxic-hypercapnic (lower response) backgrounds. Approximate inspired PCO_2 andPO_2 of each gas mixture are indicated. Note that the first significant drop in ventilation occurred at breath 3 during hypoxia and at breath 5 during hyperoxia, consistent with hyperoxia inactivating the peripheral chemoreceptors. (Modified from Miller *et al.* (1974). 'The transient respiratory effects in man of sudden changes in alveolar CO_2 in hypoxia and in high oxygen.' *Respiration Physiology* 20, 17–31.)

(b) cerebral hyperperfusion caused by the low P_aO_2 (Kety & Schmidt, 1948) which would reduce cerebral PCO_2 and the central chemoreceptor drive to $\dot{V}_E$. The increase of cerebral blood flow with hypoxia is apparent at a higher P_aO_2 than the cerebral acidosis (Javaheri, 1986).

Middle Range (P_aO_2 ca. 80–200 mmHg or 10.7–26.7 kPa).
As noted above, there is no firm consensus regarding the degree and duration of hypoxic exposure required to evoke $\dot{V}_E$

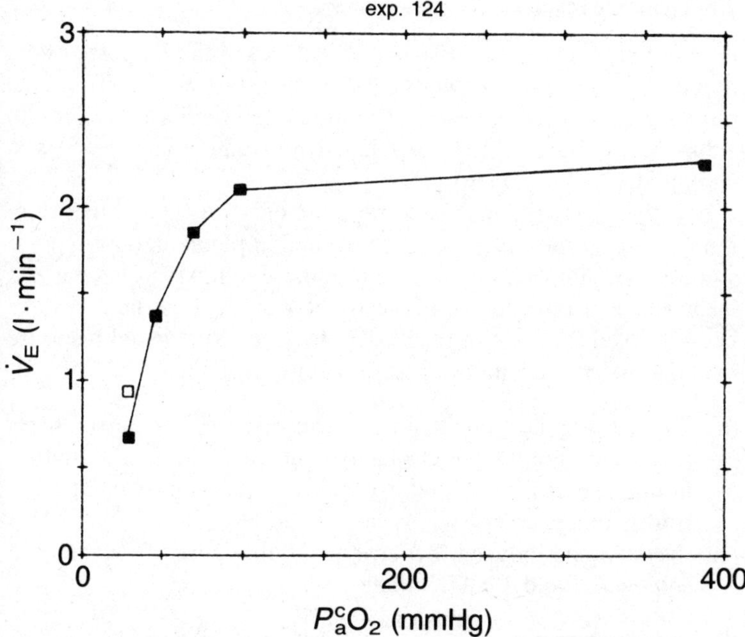

Fig. 2.4 Steady-state ventilatory ($\dot{V}_E$) response as a function of arteral P_{O2} of blood perfusing the brain stem ($P_a^cO_2$) in an anaesthetised cat undergoing separate controlled perfusion of the central and peripheral choreceptor regions. $P_a^cO_2$ was 46 mmHg; arterial PO_2 and PCO_2 at the peripheral chemoreceptors were 380 and 58 mmHg, respectively. Measurements were made starting from the lowest PO_2 and ending at the highest (■); subsequently, a single further measurement was made at low PO_a (□). (From Beck *et al.* (1984). 'Effects of brainstem hypoxaemia on the regulation of breathing.' *Respiration Physiology* 57, 171–88.)

depression. Some investigators (see Lahiri & Gelfand, 1981) have argued that the phenomenon occurs with relatively modest degrees of hypoxia (i.e. P_aO_2 ca. 80 mmHg or 10.7 kPa). Support for this contention comes from experiments on cats with separate, controlled brainstem perfusion in which mild reductions of PO_2 in the perfusate caused a fall of $\dot{V}_E$ (van Beek *et al.*, 1984) (Figure 2.4). If this is also the case in man, then conventional estimates of the hypoxic sensitivity (see below) may well underestimate the contribution of the carotid bodies.

2.5 **Dynamic response characteristics**

As a detailed review of the dynamic features of the $\dot{V}_E$ response to hypoxia is beyond the scope of this chapter, we shall confine ourselves to a brief overview. The interested reader is referred to Whipp & Wiberg (1983), Benchetrit & Demongeot (1986) and Cunningham *et al.* (1986).

In general terms, many of the engineers' test functions (e.g. impulse, step, ramp, sinusoid) have been implemented as hypoxic stimuli. The simplest way to generate these in man has been in the inspired gas, from which useful estimates of response latency have been derived (e.g. Dejours, 1962). However, the actual response dynamics of $\dot{V}_E$ are more difficult to interpret since:

(a) the PO_2 step is attenuated in its transmission from inspired gas to arterial blood owing to factors such as mixing and dilution in lung gas stores and heterogeneity of pulmonary circulatory transit times; and
(b) the hypoxia-induced hyperpnoea will cause P_aO_2 to rise somewhat, and P_aCO_2 to fall.

The resulting stimulus profile presented to the carotid bodies and central chemoreceptors will be quite complex.

In an attempt to overcome some of these difficulties, both manual and computerised techniques have been implemented for generating specific dynamic profiles of alveolar gas tensions in man by continuous control of the corresponding inspired tensions (Figure 2.2). These approaches have yielded a largely linear, first-order $\dot{V}_E$ response to $P_{ET}O_2$ steps (Swanson *et al.*, 1978; Gardner, 1980); although the response to isocapnic sinusoids of hypoxia suggests that the dynamics may be more complex and incorporate an element of rate sensitivity (Robbins, 1984). The carotid chemoreceptor discharge in animals appears to possess similar dynamic features (see Whipp *et al.*, 1983; Fitzgerald & Lahiri, 1986); although the $\dot{V}_E$ dynamics (with a time constant of ca. 10–16 s: Gardner, 1980) are an order of magnitude slower. This may reflect both a degree of alveolar-to-arterial attenuation of the hypoxic signal (see above) and central neural processing of the kind described by Eldridge (1974), for example, in which the abrupt removal of a carotid body stimulus in the cat was manifest as a slow decay of ventilatory activity rather than an immediate and abrupt decrease; however, it is unclear to what extent this mechanism normally contributes to hypoxic ventilatory response dynamics in man.

2.6 **Modulators of hypoxic sensitivity**

A variety of factors have been shown to influence hypoxic sensitivity in man. We confine ourselves here, however, to consideration of a few of the more common examples pertinent to the normal operation of the ventilatory control system.

CO_2-H^+
The $\dot{V}_E$ response to hypoxia has been widely shown to be potentiated by increases in $P_{ET}CO_2$ (reviewed by Cunningham, 1974 and Rebuck & Slutsky, 1981) (Figure 2.1). The potentiation, implicit in the steepening of the $\dot{V}_E$-$P_{ET}CO_2$ relationship by hypoxia (Nielsen & Smith, 1952), appears to take place at the carotid bodies rather than more centrally within the brainstem (Swanson *et al.*, 1978; Cunningham *et al.*, 1986) (Figure 2.2).

Exercise
Hypoxia augments the magnitude of exercise hyperpnoea considerably, through actions which appear to involve primarily the carotid bodies (see Chapter 5 for detailed discussion).

Catecholamines
Various catecholamines which occur naturally within the carotid bodies have been shown to influence carotid chemoreceptor discharge (reviewed by McDonald, 1981) and $\dot{V}_E$. Thus, noradrenaline can increase hypoxic sensitivity (reviewed by Lloyd & Cunningham, 1963 and Cunningham, 1974). In contrast, dopamine (an inhibitory neurotransmitter at the carotid bodies) reduces hypoxic sensitivity (Welsh *et al.*, 1978; Ward & Bellville, 1982).

Temperature
Hyperthermia can increase $\dot{V}_E$ in man, through probably a complex interplay of factors (metabolic rate, chemoreceptors, central

respiratory neurones). In the cat, there is evidence of an increased hypoxic sensitivity of carotid chemoreceptors (Lahiri & Gelfand, 1981) which is consistent with the increased $\dot{V}_E$ sensitivity to hypoxia reported by Petersen & Vejby-Christensen (1977) in man during hyperthermia.

2.7 Methods for assessing hypoxic sensitivity

The satisfactory characterisation of a subject's steady-state $\dot{V}_E$-$P_{ET}O_2$ relationship requires the imposition of a range of different inhaled O_2 fractions (Figure 2.1), each for sufficient time to allow a new steady-state $\dot{V}_E$ to develop (typically a few minutes under isocapnic conditions: Figure 2.2). If $P_{ET}CO_2$ is not held stable, this requirement may be prolonged as the central chemoreceptors adjust to an altered level of stimulation. Thus, the procedure may become time-consuming and stressful for the subject. Expedients have therefore been proposed in an attempt to reduce the time required for such estimations.

One approach which reduces the data density required for estimations of hypoxic sensitivity depends on the prior assumption of certain parameter values. For example, for the hyperbolic expression of eqn (2.2), parameter C may be held constant so that only A' requires estimation (Weil *et al.*, 1971); this can, however, bias the estimation significantly (Cunningham, 1974; Rebuck & Slutsky, 1981).

An alternative approach, now widely used in clinical situations, relies on a dynamic method for estimating hypoxic sensitivity. Rebuck & Campbell (1974) have developed a rebreathing (i.e. non-steady-state) method for imposing progressive isocapnic hypoxia. This approach is analogous to the Read CO_2 rebreathing technique (see Chapter 3) in that, while steady-state conditions are never actually attained in the test, the $\dot{V}_E$ response to the hypoxia will (after a short delay phase at the start of the test) develop at the same rate as in the steady-state. This technique enables a greater density of data to be obtained over a shorter time interval. Careful design of the CO_2-absorbing system coupled with manual dexterity are necessary to ensure isocapnia, however. Regardless of technique, it is advisable to limit the duration of hypoxic episodes where possible, in view of the potential drawback of hypoxic depression (see above).

Mention should also be made of the transient O_2-switching technique of Dejours (1962). While this does not furnish a rigorously validated parameter of hypoxic sensitivity, it may provide a useful index of the carotid body contribution to $\dot{V}_E$ and is also simple to implement: with a delay of 2–3 breaths (consistent with the lung-to-carotid body transit time), the abrupt and surreptitious replacement of air with 100% O_2 evokes a transient fall of $\dot{V}_E$ which continues for 20–25 s. This response has been ascribed to carotid body inactivation as it cannot be discerned in carotid-body-resected subjects (Whipp & Wasserman, 1980). The magnitude of the transient fall in $\dot{V}_E$ is taken to reflect the eupnoeic carotid body contribution to $\dot{V}_E$; under certain conditions, however, other factors may complicate this simple interpretation (see Whipp *et al.*, 1983, for detailed discussion).

In conclusion, while the ventilatory response to hypoxia in man primarily reflects the activity of the carotid chemoreceptors, interpretations regarding hypoxic sensitivity should also take account of factors related to the central neural consequences of extreme hyperoxia and hypoxia and to factors which modulate carotid chemoreceptor sensitivity. A further complicating feature is that impairments in the carotid chemo-reflex loop may occur downstream of the receptor (as in some pulmonary disease states and high-pressure environments) and thus compromise the flow-generating capability of the respiratory system. The $\dot{V}_E$-$P_{ET}O_2$ relationship should therefore be regarded as an overall input-output characteristic of the human ventilatory control system.

2.8 **Further reading**

Cunningham, D. J. C., Robbins, P. A. & Wolff, C. B. (1986). Integration of respiratory responses to changes in alveolar partial pressures of CO_2 and O_2 and in arterial pH. In: *Handbook of Physiology, Sect. 3. The Respiratory System, vol. 2.* (Cherniack, N. S. & Widdicombe, J. G., eds.), pp. 475–528. American Physiological Society, Washington, D.C.

Lahiri, S. & Gelfand, R. (1981). Mechanisms of acute ventilatory responses. In *Regulation of Breathing, part II* (Hornbein, T. F., ed.), pp. 773–843. Dekker, New York.

Rebuck, A. S. & Slutsky, A. S. (1981). Measurement of

ventilatory responses to hypercapnia and hypoxia. In: *Regulation of Breathing, part II*, (Hornbein, T. F., ed.), pp. 745–71. Dekker, New York.

Whipp, B. J., Wasserman, K. & Ward, S. A. (1983). Reflex control of ventilation by peripheral arterial chemoreceptors in man. In: *Physiology of the Peripheral Arterial Chemoreceptors.* (Acker, H. & O'Regan, R. G., eds.), pp. 299–323. Elsevier, Amsterdam.

References

Beek, J. H. G. M. van, Berkenbosch, A., DeGoede, J. & Olievier, C. N. (1984). Effects of brainstem hypoxaemia on the regulation of breathing. *Respiration Physiology*, **57**, 171–88.

Benchetrit, G. & Demongeot, J., eds. (1987). *Concepts and Formalizations in the Control of Breathing.* Manchester University Press, Manchester.

Cherniack, N. S., Edelman, N. H. & Lahiri, S. (1971). Hypoxia and hypercapnia as respiratory stimulants and depressants. *Respiration Physiology*, **11**, 113–26.

Cunningham, D. J. C. (1974). Integrative aspects of the regulation of breathing: A personal view. In: *MTP International Review of Science* (Guyton, A. C. & Widdicombe, J. G., eds.) pp. 303–69. University Park Press, Baltimore.

Cunningham, D. J. C., Robbins, P. A. & Wolff, C. B. (1986). Integration of respiratory responses to changes in alveolar partial pressures of CO_2 and O_2 and in arterial pH. In: *Handbook of Physiology, Sect. 3. The Respiratory System, vol. 2.* (Cherniack, N. S. & Widdicombe, J. G., eds.), pp. 475–528. American Physiological Society, Washington, D.C.

Dautrebande, L. & Haldane, J. S. (1922). The effects of respiration of oxygen on breathing and circulation. *Journal of Physiology*, **55**, 296–9.

Dejours, P. (1962). Chemoreflexes in breathing. *Physiological Reviews*, **42**, 335–58.

Eldridge, F. L. (1974). Central neural respiratory stimulatory effects of active respiration. *Journal of Applied Physiology*, **37**, 723–735.

Fitzgerald, R. S. & Lahiri, S. (1986). Reflex responses to chemoreceptor stimulation. In: *Handbook of Physiology, Sect. 3. The Respiratory System, vol. 2.* (Cherniack, N. S. & Widdicombe, J. G. eds.) pp. 313–62. American Physiological Society, Washington, D.C.

Gardner, W. N. (1980). The pattern of breathing following step changes of alveolar partial pressures of carbon dioxide and oxygen. *Journal of Physiology*, **300**, 55–73.

Guz, A., Noble M. I. M., Widdicombe, J. G., Trenchard, D. & Mushin, W. W. (1966). Peripheral chemoreceptor block in man. *Respiration Physiology*, **1**, 38–40.

Honda, Y., Watanabe, S., Hashizume, I., Satomura, Y., Hata, N.,

Sakakibara, Y. & Severinghaus, J. W. (1979). Hypoxic chemosensitivity in asthmatic patients two decades after carotid body resection. *Journal of Applied Physiology*, **46**, 632–38.

Jahaveri, S. (1986). Hypoxia lowers cerebrovascular resistance without changing brain and blood pH. *Journal of Applied Physiology*, **60**, 802–8.

Kety, S. S. & Schmidt, C. F. (1948). The effects of altered arterial tensions of carbon dioxide and oxygen on cerebral blood flow and cerebral oxygen consumption of normal young men. *Journal of Clinical Investigation*, **27**, 484–95.

Kronenberg, R., Hamilton, F. N., Gabel, R., Hickey, R., Read, D. J. C. & Severinghaus, J. (1973). Comparison of three methods for quantitating respiratory response to hypoxia in man. *Respiration Physiology*, **16**, 109–25.

Lahiri, S. & Gelfand, R. (1981). Mechanisms of acute ventilatory responses. In: *Regulation of Breathing, part II* (Hornbein, T. F., ed.), pp. 773–843. Dekker, New York.

Lambertsen, C. J., Kough, R. H., Cooper, D. Y., Emmel, G. L., Loeschcke, H. H. & Schmidt, C. F. (1953). Comparison of relationship of respiratory minute volume to P_{CO2} and pH of arterial and internal jugular blood in normal man during hyperventilation produced by low concentrations of CO_2 at 1 atmosphere and by O_2 at 3.0 atmospheres. *Journal of Applied Physiology*, **5**, 803–13.

Lloyd, B. B. & Cunningham, D. J. C. (1963). Quantitative approach to the regulation of human respiration. In: *The Regulation of Human Respiration*, (Cunningham, D. J. C. & Lloyd, B. B., eds.) pp. 331–49. Blackwell, Oxford.

McDonald, D. M. (1981). Peripheral chemoreceptors: structure-function relationships in the carotid body. In: *Regulation of Breathing, part I*, (Hornbein, T. F., ed.), pp. 105–319. Dekker, New York.

Miller, J. D., Cunningham, D. J. C., Lloyd, B. B. & Young, J. M. (1974). The transient respiratory effects in man of sudden changes in alveolar CO_2 in hypoxia and in high oxygen. *Respiration Physiology*, **20**, 17–31.

Nielsen, M. & Smith, H. (1952). Studies on the regulation of respiration in acute hypoxia. *Acta Physiologica Scandinavica*, **24**, 293–313.

Petersen, E. S. & Vejby-Christensen, H. (1977). Effects of body temperature on ventilatory response to hypoxia and breathing pattern in man. *Journal of Applied Physiology*, **42**, 492–500.

Ponten, U. & Siesjo, B. K. (1966). Gradients of CO_2 tension in the brain. *Acta Physiologica Scandinavica*, **67**, 129–40.

Rebuck, A. S. & Campbell, E. J. M. (1974). A clinical method for assessing the ventilatory response to hypoxia. *American Review of Respiratory Disease*, **109**, 345–50.

Rebuck, A. S. & Slutsky, A. S. (1981). Measurement of ventilatory responses to hypercapnia and hypoxia. In: *Regulation of Breathing, part II*, (Hornbein, T. F., ed.), pp. 745–71. Dekker, New York.

Robbins, P. A. (1984). The ventilatory response of the human respiratory system to sine waves of alveolar carbon dioxide and hypoxia. *Journal of Physiology*, **350**, 461–474.

Saunders, N. A., Powles, A. C. P. & Rebuck, A. S. (1976). Ear oximetry: Accuracy and practicability in the assessment of arterial oxygenation. *American Review of Respiratory Disease*, **113**, 745–9.

Severinghaus, J. W. (1976). Proposed standard determination of ventilatory responses to hypoxia and hypercapnia in man. *Chest*, **70** (suppl.), 129–31.

Siesjo, B. K., Johannsson, H., Norberg, K. & Salford, L. (1975). Brain function metabolism and blood flow in moderate and severe arterial hypoxia. In: *Brain Work*, (Ingvar, D. H. & Lassen, N. A., eds.), pp. 101–9. Munksgaard, Copenhagen.

Swanson, G. D., Whipp, B. J., Kaufman, R. D., Aqleh, K. A., Winter, B. & Bellville, J. W. (1978). Effect of hypercapnia on hypoxic ventilatory drive in normal and carotid body-resected man. *Journal of Applied Physiology*, **45**, 971–7.

Ward, D. S. & Bellville, J. W. (1982). Reduction of hypoxic ventilatory drive by dopamine. *Anesthesia and Analgesia*, **61**, 333–7.

Ward, S. A. & Bellville, J. W. (1983). Peripheral chemoreflex suppression by hyperoxia during moderate exercise in man. In: *Modelling and Control of Breathing*, (Whipp, B. J. & Wiberg, D. M., eds), pp. 54–61. Elsevier, New York.

Weil, J. V., Byrne-Quinne, E., Sodal, I. E., Filley, G. F. & Grover, R. F. (1971). Acquired attenuation of chemoreceptor function in chronically hypoxic man at high altitude. *Journal of Clinical Investigation*, **50**, 186–95.

Weil, J. V., Byrne-Quinne, E., Sodal, I. E., Friesen, W. O, Underhill, B., Filley, G. F. & Grover, R. F. (1970). Hypoxic ventilatory drive in normal man. *Journal of Clinical Investigation*, **49**, 1061–72.

Welsh, M. J., Heistad, D. D. & Abboud, F. M. (1978). Effect of dopamine on ventilation in man. *Journal of Clinical Investigation*, **61**, 708–13.

Whipp, B. J. & Wasserman, K. (1980). Carotid bodies and ventilatory control dynamics in man. *Federation Proceedings*, **39**, 2668–73.

Whipp, B. J., Wasserman, K. & Ward, S. A. (1983). Reflex control of ventilation by peripheral arterial chemoreceptors in man. In: *Physiology of the Peripheral Arterial Chemoreceptors*. (Acker, H. & O'Regan, R. G., eds.), pp. 299–323. Elsevier, Amsterdam.

Whipp, B. J. & Wiberg, D. M., eds. (1983). *Modelling and Control of Breathing*. Elsevier, New York.

3

The ventilatory response to inhaled CO_2

R. C. Cummin and K. B. Saunders Department of Medicine 1, St. George's Hospital Medical School, London

3.1 **Introduction**

In 1905 Haldane & Priestley demonstrated that the respiratory system is very sensitive to perturbations of alveolar PCO_2 (P_ACO_2) and that, in any one individual, P_ACO_2 is remarkably constant. While many factors are now known to play a part in the control of ventilation ($\dot{V}_E$), the relative constancy of mean alveolar and arterial PCO_2 (P_aCO_2) both at rest and during moderate exercise suggests a pivotal role for CO_2. Interest has therefore continued in the relationship between $\dot{V}_E$ and P_ACO_2 or P_aCO_2; this is sometimes referred to as the **CO_2 response**. Although P_ACO_2 or P_aCO_2 and $\dot{V}_E$ are the usually estimated variables, it is worth noting at the outset that while these are not ideal measures of either the input or the output of the ventilatory control system, the CO_2 response has the advantage of being easy to obtain and clinically applicable.

3.2 **Steady-State methods**

CO_2 responses were originally obtained by measuring the steady-state $\dot{V}_E$ and P_ACO_2 (i.e. end-tidal) of a subject breathing a series of gases with differing values of PCO_2 (Nielsen & Smith, 1952; Lloyd *et al.*, 1958). One problem with this approach is that the load of CO_2 delivered to the subject increases as $\dot{V}_E$ rises, so that the steady state is delayed. Some 20 min may thus be required to determine each point on the response curve, which makes the method tedious and unpleasant for the subject. That the delay is partly a feature of the method of CO_2 administration can be demonstrated with computer models and has been confirmed experimentally (Saunders *et al.*, 1980*a* and *b*).

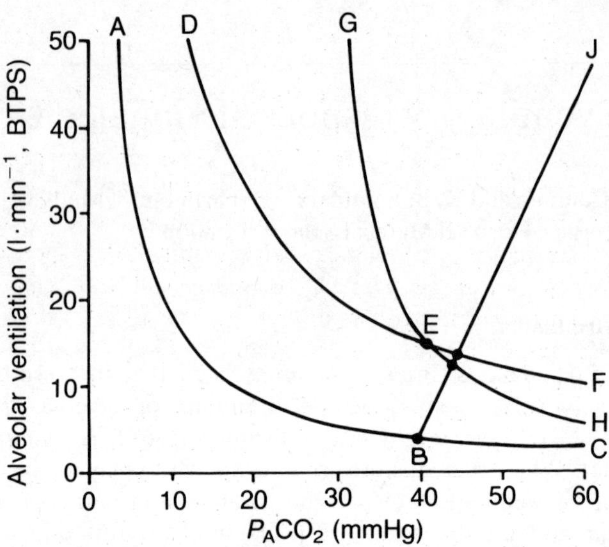

Fig. 3.1 The metabolic hyperbola for a $\dot{V}_{CO_2}$ of $0.2\,l \cdot min^{-1}$ (ABC) and for a $\dot{V}_{CO_2}$ of $0.8\,l \cdot min^{-1}$ (DEF) breathing air, and the metabolic hyperbola for a $\dot{V}_{CO_2}$ of $0.2\,l \cdot min^{-1}$ breathing 4% CO_2-in-air (GEH). At $\dot{V}_A = 15\,l \cdot min^{-1}$, the total CO_2 load is the same for DEF and GEH at point E. BJ is a CO_2 response line. (Modified from Fenn & Craig, 1963).

With the classical method, the presence of a fixed inspired PCO_2 (P_ICO_2) impairs the clearance of CO_2 by the increased $\dot{V}_E$. As shown in Figure 3.1, for air-breathing subjects the steady-state alveolar ventilation ($\dot{V}_A$) and P_ACO_2 lie on a hyperbola (ABC) described by the Alveolar Air Equation. With an increased P_ICO_2, however, this hyperbola is shifted to the right such that the asymptote lies at the new P_ICO_2 (GEH). Steady-state $\dot{V}_A$ and P_ACO_2 are represented by the point at which the CO_2 response line (BJ) crosses the hyperbola. Note that the gradient of the hyperbola GEH at this point is much steeper than the hyperbola DEF which is the hyperbola for exercise at the same PCO_2. Thus, with a fixed P_ICO_2, larger changes in $\dot{V}_A$ are required for a given change in P_ACO_2. Furthermore, whatever the subject's $\dot{V}_A$, P_ACO_2 can never be lower than that of the inspired gas. With a low P_ICO_2, it would be possible for a sensitive control system to return P_ACO_2 to, or near to, normal; with higher values of P_ICO_2, however, this would require a $\dot{V}_A$ response which approaches infinity as P_ICO_2 approaches P_ACO_2.

Because of the increased difficulty in clearing CO_2 when P_ICO_2 is fixed and elevated, it was thought possible that the respiratory centre might tolerate a higher PCO_2 than would have been the case if the hyperbola had been similar to that found in exercise. Fenn & Craig (1963) even considered whether this might account for the discrepancy between the classical resting CO_2 response and the situation in exercise when $\dot{V}_E$ increases with little change in P_aCO_2. To test this hypothesis, they performed CO_2 responses which mimicked the hyperbola of exercise by fixing the inspiratory CO_2 load. This was done by injecting pure CO_2 into the inspiratory air stream at a constant flow: the subject's CO_2 load was kept constant whatever the $\dot{V}_E$. They found no difference in the resting CO_2 responses whether CO_2 was administered as a constant concentration or as a constant inflow.

Fenn & Craig's technique does have some important practical advantages. Because the CO_2 load does not depend on $\dot{V}_E$ and normal feedback relationships and maintained, the steady state is reached more rapidly (Saunders *et al.*, 1980b). Further, small CO_2 loads can be delivered with precision and these are not affected by the increasing $\dot{V}_E$ during exercise.

3.3 **The Rebreathing method**

The length of time required to achieve steady-state CO_2 responses using a series of P_ICO_2 values led to a search for a more rapid alternative suitable for clinical use. It was soon realised that an estimate of CO_2 sensitivity could be obtained from a subject's response to breathing in and out of a bag: the PCO_2 in the bag gradually rises, as does $\dot{V}_E$; there is no steady state. The method has been progressively refined so that, by starting with a small bag containing gas with a PCO_2 close to mixed venous ($P_{\bar{v}}CO_2$), an equilibrium is reached rapidly and the PCO_2 in the bag rises linearly with time with very little transfer of CO_2 to the bag (Read, 1967). The PCO_2 in the bag, in mixed venous blood and at the chemoreceptors are in equilibrium and rise together. The bag PCO_2 is very close to, and can be taken to represent, the PCO_2 at the chemoreceptors. Hypoxia is avoided by starting with a high PO_2 in the bag.

Unlike the other methods, rebreathing completely abolishes the normal within-breath P_aCO_2 oscillations (see Chapter 4). This can be an advantage as it allows the system to be studied free of any signals that may be derived from the oscillations. A more obvious disadvantage stems from the high starting PCO_2 which, of necessity, is near to $P_{\bar{v}}CO_2$; thus, only the physiologically least interesting top part of the CO_2 response can be studied.

Using steady-state methods the feedback loop between $\dot{V}_E$ and chemoreceptor PCO_2 is preserved although, when CO_2 is administered at a constant concentration, the relationship is altered such that larger changes in $\dot{V}_E$ are required to alter PCO_2 (Figure 3.1). In contrast, when the rebreathing technique is used, provided that the bag is small enough, $\dot{V}_E$ cannot alter chemoreceptor PCO_2 and the feedback loop is broken.

The rebreathing method is often applied in clinical situations because it is simple, quick, well-tolerated and P_ACO_2 can be taken to represent P_aCO_2 even in conditions of ventilation-perfusion mismatch. However, the agreement between the rebreathing and steady-state methods does not apply under conditions of metabolic acid-base disturbance (Linton *et al.*, 1973). With the classical steady-state method, metabolic acidosis and alkalosis shift the intercept of the CO_2 response curve but the slope is unchanged. With the rebreathing method, the results are quite different: the slope is increased with metabolic acidosis and decreased with metabolic alkalosis, but the intercept is unaffected. The reasons for these discrepancies are unclear, and thus it cannot be said that either method is more or less valid with alterations in acid-base status.

Problems may also arise if rebreathing is used in exercise when rapid shrinkage of the bag due to the high O_2 consumption may alter the linearity of the rise in PCO_2.

3.4 **Dynamic responses**

Steady-state responses give information about linearity and overall gain, but do not allow us to predict what the time course of the $\dot{V}_E$ response will be to a given CO_2 input; the dynamic response must be otained. This is done by a variety of forcing techniques (see Chapter 1 section 1.10).

3.4.1 *Sinusoid*

Stoll (1969) imposed a sinusoidally-changing P_ICO_2 at various frequencies in man, and analysed the results as a second order system: one component had a short time delay of a few seconds and a time constant of about 30 s, and the other had a similar pure time delay but a much larger time constant (ca. 400 s); both components contributed about equally to the overall gain. It was tempting to ascribe these two components respectively to the peripheral and central chemoreceptors. This was achieved by Daubenspeck (1973) who used a similar second order analysis in the cat: the faster component (which contributed in this case only about one-fifth of the overall gain) disappeared after cutting the carotid sinus nerve. Swanson & Bellville (1974) improved the technique by using feedback methods to produce sinusoidal variations in end-tidal PCO_2($P_{ET}CO_2$) and PO_2 ($P_{ET}O_2$). Their work yielded important evidence regarding the location of the interaction between hypoxic and hypercapnic stimuli in man (see below).

3.4.2 *Steps changes*

Swanson & Bellville (1975) and Chambille *et al.* (1975) developed this technique in man, again by the use of feedback control of inspired gas tensions. A second order analysis again gave gains, time delays and time constants which seemed appropriate for the central and peripheral chemoreceptors. As always, in man, it is a large assumption to ascribe two analytically defined components to two anatomically and physiologically separate structures. DeGoede *et al.* (1985) provided most important evidence towards this point by comparing, in cats, the dynamic forcing technique of Swanson & Bellville (1975) with their own technique of separately perfusing the central and peripheral chemoreceptors and thus isolating the separate chemoreceptor dynamic responses. There was good correspondence between dynamic forcing and differential perfusion in terms of gains and time constants, giving strong support to the overall validity of the non-invasive dynamic forcing technique.

3.4.3 *Brief stimuli*

This subject is reviewed by Dejours (1962) and Cunningham

(1974). The potential advantages of single-breath or similarly brief stimuli are that:

(a) small stimuli should produce small $\dot{V}_E$ responses, perhaps unnoticeable to the subject, which minimise any conscious attempt of the subject to adjust breathing;
(b) cerebral blood flow is likely to be unaltered by brief PCO_2 transients.

The disadvantages are that small $\dot{V}_E$ responses are difficult to detect against a noisy baseline and thus Bouverot *et al.* (1965) used two breaths of 7% CO_2; however, this level can be detected as an acid taste by many subjects. This disadvantage can be overcome by suddenly reducing a moderately high P_ICO_2 to zero; an approach which was exploited by Miller *et al.* (1974) in man to show different $\dot{V}_E$ response latencies for the peripheral and central chemoreceptors (*ca.* two and five breaths, respectively). A further disadvantage is that without precise description of both input and output (which is difficult to obtain with small stimuli) it is not possible to determine the overall gains or time constants of a response, even though the pure time delays are detectable. Thus, comparison with results from steady-state techniques is difficult.

3.5 **Measurement of input**

It is PCO_2 which is taken to be the stimulus to both the peripheral and central chemoreceptors, though there is controversy about whether this acts directly or via changes in $[H^+]$. Both P_ACO_2 and P_aCO_2 oscillate with breathing, rising during expiration and falling during inspiration: the amplitude of these oscillations is calculated to be about 2–3 mmHg at rest (depending on breathing frequency) and to rise with increasing work load on exercise to as much as 10–15 mmHg (1.3–2.0 kPa) (see Chapter 4). At rest, it is accepted that $P_{ET}CO_2$ is a reasonable approximation to mean (time-averaged) P_ACO_2; i.e. it is sampled from towards the top of the P_ACO_2 oscillation. During exercise, however, $P_{ET}CO_2$ is still sampled from towards the peak, but – as the oscillation is steeper – it may be 5 mmHg (0.7 kPa) above mean P_ACO_2. This has made it difficult to assess the CO_2 response during exercise. The problem is shown schematically in Figure 3.2 where the PCO_2 record at

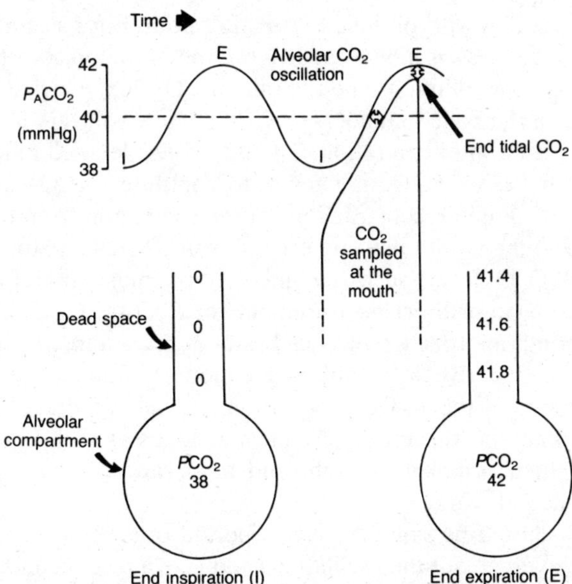

Fig. 3.2 Diagramatic representation of a respiratory-related alveolar PCO_2 oscillation during light exercise (amplitude 4 mmHg or 0.5 kPa), top; the PCO_2 in a simple lung model at end-inspiration (I), bottom left, and at end-expiration (E), bottom right. The record of CO_2 sampled at the mouth (top right) is displaced to the right, and end-tidal PCO_2 is less than maximum alveolar PCO_2.

the mouth is displaced in time to the right by the transport delay between alveolus and mouth, and $P_{ET}CO_2$ is therefore less than the maximum P_ACO_2 since the highest alveolar value is never seen at the mouth because of the flow reversal. However, the magnitude of the difference (Figure 3.2) is likely to be small.

One approach to this problem is to attempt a reconstruction of the P_ACO_2 oscillation from a time-average of the recording at the mouth (DuBois *et al.*, 1952; Ward & Whipp, 1980). However, this cannot be done accurately because the peak of the oscillation is never seen, and also because the time course of P_ACO_2 in the earliest part of inspiration just after point E (Figure 3.2) is not easily predictable. The early inspirate is from the dead space (Figure 3.2, bottom right) which has a marginally lower PCO_2. If the continuing CO_2 transfer is faster than this weak inspiratory dilution, P_ACO_2 will continue to rise after point E for a short time. Whether it does or not depends on the initial magnitude of inspiratory flow (dilution) and the rate of CO_2 flux, which is low at this stage of the cycle (Saunders *et al.*, 1980) and will vary inversely with the duration of expiration. Thus, a rather detailed modelling of alveolar gas exchange is needed to compute P_ACO_2 in early inspiration; simple reconstructions of the oscillation from tracings recorded at the mouth being in error to some extent. Estimates of mean P_ACO_2 from such reconstructions must therefore be calibrated against direct measurements of P_aCO_2.

A second approach is to calibrate P_ACO_2 directly against $P_{ET}CO_2$ and derive a suitable regression equation. The major determinants of the P_ACO_2 oscillation are mean metabolic rate, tidal volume and respiratory frequency. Jones *et al.* (1979) have derived such formulae for light and moderate exercise, a most useful piece of work.

P_aCO_2 should be sampled over a period of several respiratory cycles to average out the oscillations and give a true mean P_aCO_2. Calibrations of reconstruction methods against P_aCO_2, and the formulae of Jones *et al.* (1979) refer only to steady-state conditions, therefore. We have no method of assessing mean P_ACO_2 or P_aCO_2 during exercise transients, nor shall we have until a suitably fast-responding CO_2 electrode is developed. This is why the dynamics of the CO_2 response are now well studied in man at rest, but not during exercise.

3.6 **Measurement of output**

The output of the respiratory centre – or **neural drive** – is best expressed in the phrenic neurogram, but in man it is $\dot{V}_E$ which is normally taken as the output. This is fair if respiratory mechanics are normal. However, if the subject has severe airflow obstruction or abnormally stiff lungs, the $\dot{V}_E$ achieved will not accurately reflect the neural drive. Some measure of **mechanical effort**, rather than mechanical achievement, is then required. **Mouth occlusion pressure** – the pressure at the mouth at 0.1 s in early inspiration during brief occlusion of the airway ($P_{0.\bar{I}}$) is the variable most frequently used (Whitelaw *et al.*, 1975; Gelb *et al.*, 1977).

It is also useful and important separately to consider the

components of the respiratory cycle: inspiratory time (T_I), expiratory time (T_E), total time or breath duration ($T_{tot} = T_I + T_E$), and tidal volume (V_T). In particular, the **mean inspiratory flow** (V_T/T_I) may be a closer reflection of neural drive than the normally calculated breath-by-breath $\dot{V}_E$ (V_T/T_{tot}). In this review we will consider only the effect of CO_2 on total (or occasionally alveolar) ventilation.

3.7 Theoretical and practical problems in performing CO_2 response measurement

3.7.1 *Changes taking place while the response is being performed*

It is dangerous to assume that while the measurement of the CO_2 response is being performed all other stimuli which might affect respiration remain constant, especially when a complete CO_2 steady-state response takes considerable time to achieve. Here the more rapid rebreathing technique has the advantage. On the other hand, the slower steady-state method allows the order in which the points are determined to be altered, and this may enable time-related influences to be detected. This is not, of course, possible with the rebreathing technique. Subjects should be seated comfortably, isolated as far as possible from apparatus and experimenters. Taped music or reading may be used to distract the subject from environmental events, but may themselves influence breathing.

3.7.2 *Linearity*

At rest a threshold or 'dog-leg' is found in hypoxic hypocapnia (Nielsen & Smith, 1952). Whether a similar alinearity may be found near the control point during air-breathing is controversial. Anthonisen & Dhingra (1978) published provocative results suggesting that low levels of inspired CO_2 were cleared isocapnically. However, careful experiments in conscious dogs (Reischl *et al.*, 1980; Reischl & Stavert, 1982) and in the cat (Fordyce *et al.*, 1984) did not bear this out, and it is now generally agreed that low levels of inspired CO_2 are not isocapnically cleared (Dempsey & Forster, 1982). The region of CO_2 response close to the control point is rarely examined in sufficient detail to characterise any local alinearities. If alinearity is found, it is usually in the opposite

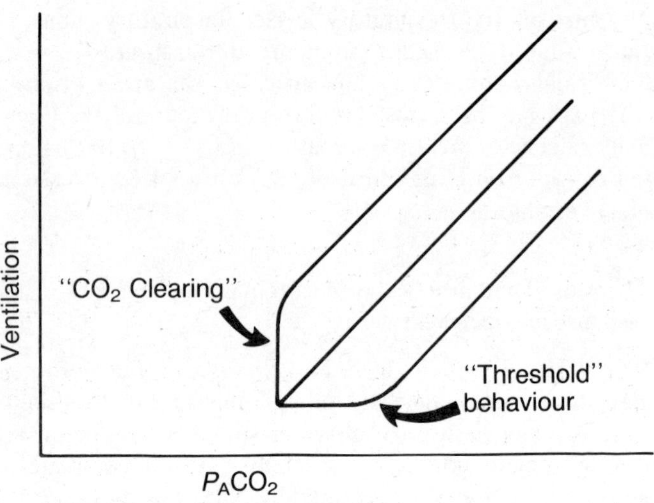

Fig. 3.3 Diagramatic representation of possible alinearities in the CO_2 response. Response with upward concavity represents a 'threshold' effect, and with downward concavity a region of 'CO_2 clearing'.

sense, with an initially low response to CO_2 (Folgering *et al.*, 1974; Forster *et al.*, 1982). If true, this implies that the CO_2 response is hardly operative during normal eucapnic breathing (Figure 3.3). However, minor hyperventilation during the control period could lead to such a flat early phase in the CO_2 response.

During exercise, there is recent evidence that the slope of the CO_2 response close to the control point may increase as work load increases (Hulsbosch *et al.*, 1982; Cummin *et al.*, 1986), giving alinearity which is concave down (Figure 3.3). These are controversial points.

3.7.3 *The effect of nose-clip and mouthpiece*

Some such apparatus is required to give controlled quantities of CO_2 by inhalation and all experiments are to the same extent contaminated by the slightly abnormal breathing which is known to be caused thereby. CO_2 can be given by a hood with a bias-flow system or in an environmental chamber, but it is then not possible to produce rapidly and precisely controlled changes in P_ACO_2.

There is no doubt that breathing with a nose-clip causes an increased V_T, usually about 25%. There is less agreement about changes in frequency (f), overall $\dot{V}_E$ or the subdivisions of the respiratory cycle; however, usually f decreases slightly, $\dot{V}_E$ is, if anything, increased and $P_{ET}CO_2$ – if it falls – may remain at its new level for over an hour (Hirsch & Bishop, 1982; Weissman *et al.*, 1984; Perez & Tobin, 1985).

3.7.4 *The influence of cerebral blood flow*

It is reasonable to take P_aCO_2 as the relevant stimulus at the carotid body, but at the central chemoreceptors it must be brain tissue PCO_2 which is the relevant variable (again, we do not enter the controversy whether PCO_2 acts directly or via local pH changes, or both). If cerebral blood flow increases, brain tissue PCO_2 will fall even if P_aCO_2 is constant. P_aCO_2 is under these circumstances a misleading variable to take as input. Much of the relevant experimental work comes of necessity from the animal laboratory. Cerebral hypoxia and hypercapnia both cause an increase in total cerebral blood flow. However, the blood flow changes in the ventral medulla are greater proportionally than changes in total cerebral flow (Britton *et al.*, 1979, in dogs; Neubauer *et al.*, 1983, and Feustel *et al.*, 1984, in cats). Neubauer & Edelman (1984) showed in awake cats that the proportionally excessive increased flow to the brainstem in hypoxia was diminished by superior cervical ganglionectomy. Uneven redistribution of flow means that calculations of brain tissue PCO_2 based on measurement of total brain flow, P_aCO_2 and brain P_vCO_2 will underestimate changes in brainstem tissue PCO_2 due to changes in cerebral blood flow.

A further complication is that changes in $\dot{V}_E$ may be associated with changes in cerebral blood flow without any change in arterial blood gases. Thus, Neubauer *et al.* (1983) produced increases in $\dot{V}_E$ in cats both by electrical stimulation of hind limb muscle and by carotid nerve stimulation, and kept arterial blood gases constant. Cerebral blood flow increased, especially in the ventral medulla. These authors postulated that increased respiratory neuronal activity produces metabolites which further stimulate activity (positive feedback). The resulting increased blood flow would remove such metabolites, and thus have a stabilising (negative feedback) effect. It is interesting that Yamamoto (1980) has postulated such a local positive feedback mechanism in a purely modelling approach.

Experiments which alter cerebral blood flow primarily and

follow secondary effects on $\dot{V}_E$ (Chapman *et al.*, 1979) and on both V_E and ventral medullary pH (Neubauer *et al.*, 1985) confirm that rapid (within 5 s) and appropriate changes occur in the local chemical stimulus and in resulting $\dot{V}_E$. It is more difficult to predict the time course of cerebral blood flow changes in response to a change in blood gases. Doblar *et al* (1979) used a sinusoidal hypoxic stimulus in goats and derived a first order response in flow with a time constant of 30–40 s. A recent study of the effect of 'step' changes in P_aCO_2 in dogs (Wilson *et al.*, 1985) is more difficult to interpret since the input steps were not abrupt: the increase had a half-time of ca. 30 s. The flow response showed a pure time delay of ca. 12 s and a half-time of ca. 2 min. The response to the step decrease in P_aCO_2 was faster. It is difficult to be precise, but we can be reasonably sure that single or dual breath inputs of low PCO_2 will produce no confounding change in cerebral blood flow, and inputs lasting up to 30 s will produce a negligible change.

The important conclusion is that the effect of all CO_2 stimuli could be reviewed in the light of their possible effect on cerebral blood flow. This effect is likely to be greater than suggested by changes in total cerebral flow. If such changes occur, P_aCO_2 (or mean P_ACO_2 or $P_{ET}CO_2$) is no longer an appropriate input variable for the central chemoreceptors.

3.8 Interpretation of changes in slope of the CO_2 response

Over a wide range, the $\dot{V}_E - P_aCO_2$ relationship is linear, and the **gradient** of this line can be taken as an index of **CO_2 sensitivity**. Between normal subjects there can be a tenfold difference in this slope. This is partly because of differences in body size but, even after correcting for this, there is still a wide normal variation. This implies that the magnitude of the slope is not critical for breathing control at rest.

A simple mathematical approach explains why this is so.

The linear part of the CO_2 response can be described by the equation

$$\dot{V}_A = S \cdot (P_ACO_2 - B) \tag{3.1}$$

where S is the slope and B is the P_ACO_2 intercept.

In the steady state $\dot{V}_A$ is also related to P_ACO_2 by the Alveolar Air Equation

$$\dot{V}_A = (\dot{V}_{CO_2} \cdot K)/P_ACO_2 \tag{3.2}$$

where $\dot{V}_{CO_2}$ is the metabolic CO_2 output and K is a dimensional constant. Combining these two equations we get the quadratic

$$S \cdot P_ACO_2 - S \cdot B \cdot P_ACO_2 - \dot{V}_{CO_2} \cdot K = 0$$

Solving this for P_ACO_2 and taking the positive root gives

$$P_ACO_2 = B/2 + [B^2/4 + (K \cdot \dot{V}_{CO_2}/S)]^{1/2} \tag{3.3}$$

If some typical values are inserted into this equation: e.g., $B = 38$, $\dot{V}_{CO2} = 0.2$, $S = 2.16$, $K = 863$, then

$$P_ACO_2 = 19 + (361 + 80)^{\frac{1}{2}} = 40$$

From this equation it can be seen that, at rest, large changes in S have a relatively small effect on the value of P_ACO_2. B is the main determinant of steady-state P_ACO_2.

The same point is made graphically in Figure 3.4. Steady-state $\dot{V}_E$ is determined by the point at which the CO_2 response line crosses the hyperbola described by the Alveolar Air Equation. Even large changes in the slope of the 'response' cause only small changes in P_ACO_2, and the effect on $\dot{V}_E$ is even less because – at the normal set point – the hyperbola is approaching its asymptote.

Eqn (3.3) may be used to test the effect of slope changes at any metabolic rate or value of B. For example, doubling the slope at rest causes a fall in P_ACO_2 of only 1 mmHg (0.1 kPa) (this is the order of magnitude of many changes in slope reported as significant in the literature – see below). As $\dot{V}_{CO_2}$ increases, and B decreases, as occurs in exercise, the importance of S is magnified. For example, at $\dot{V}_{CO2}$ of $1.0 \, l \cdot min^{-1}$ (about 50 W), doubling S from 2.16 to 4.32 is responsible for a fall of 4 mmHg (0.5 kPa) if $B = 38$ mmHg (5.1 kPa), and 4.4 mmHg (0.6 kPa) if $B = 30$ mmHg (4.0 kPa).

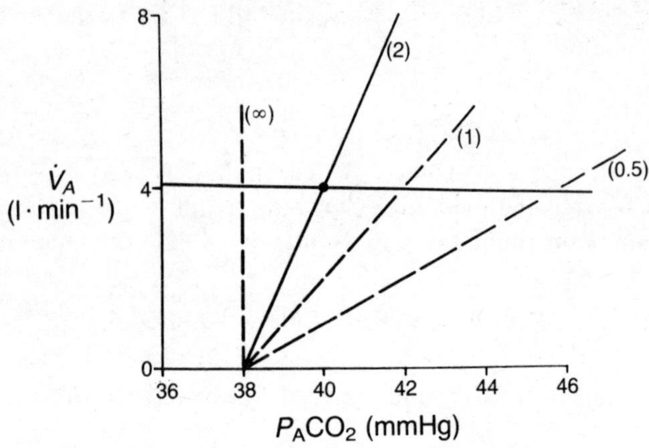

Fig. 3.4 Four CO_2 response lines of varying slope (value given in brackets) and intercept B = 38 mmHg (5.1 kPa). These lines cross the metabolic hyperbola for $\dot{V}_{CO_2}$ = 0.22 L · min^{-1}; their points of intersection define steady-state alveolar ventilation ($\dot{V}_A$) and P_ACO_2. Increasing the slope from 1.0 to infinity causes a fall in P_ACO_2 of only 4 mmHg (0.5 kPa) and a probably unmeasurable change in $\dot{V}_A$.

3.9 Central and peripheral chemoreceptors: interaction with hypoxia

Since the dynamic $P_{ET}CO_2$ forcing method used in man by Swanson & Bellville (1975) has now been validated in the animal laboratory by DeGoede *et al.* (1985), (see above), we may have added confidence in the dynamic forcing analysis. Results suggest that about 45% of the overall gain is provided by the peripheral chemoreceptors, which is a larger proportion than that previously estimated in man (Lugliani *et al.*, 1971) and greater than the value of 20% found in anaesthetised cats by DeGoede *et al.* (1985) in their comparison experiments. In man, the time constant of the first (peripheral chemoreceptor) component was about 20 s and of the slower (central chemoreceptor) component about 75 s. The response of the combined system to a step change in $P_{ET}CO_2$ reached a steady state in 5 min: this might occur earlier if a small initial overshoot were introduced into the CO_2 input wave form (Severinghaus, 1976), and this is what the constant inflow technique does (Saunders *et al.*, 1980b). The time to steady state of 5 min fits well with the similar time course of medullary extracellular pH caused by step changes of P_ICO_2 in anaesthetised cats (Eldridge *et al.*, 1984).

While it is accepted that the multiplicative interaction between hypoxia and hypercapnia (Lloyd *et al.*, 1958) occurs at the peripheral chemoreceptors (Cunningham, 1974), there is still considerable debate about the effects of hypoxia centrally and to what degree it causes central depression of respiration. There are several major obstacles:

(1) It is difficult to distinguish between a direct depressive effect of hypoxia on respiratory neuronal function and a simultaneous effect of increased cerebral perfusion that depresses $\dot{V}_E$ by washing out CO_2 (Weiskopf & Gabel, 1975).
(2) There seems to be a marked individual variation in the magnitude of any central depressant effect of hypoxia in man (Honda *et al.*, 1981).
(3) Peripheral stimulatory and central depressive effects have different time courses (Honda *et al.*, 1981). Thus, in man an initial rise in $\dot{V}_E$ may be followed by a secondary fall, making a 'steady-state' response to a given hypoxic stimulus difficult to define.
(4) A given period of hypoxia may have persisting effects on $\dot{V}_E$ and the CO_2 response. In glomectomised cats, acute severe hypoxia can cause a subsequent, prolonged (*ca.* 1 h) depression of $\dot{V}_E$ by way of a mechanism which involves the action of adenosine and can be inhibited by theophylline (Millhorn *et al.*, 1984; Eldridge *et al.*, 1985). In man, however, Davidson & Cameron (1985) found that after a 5 min period of breathing 7–8% O_2, the slope of the CO_2 response was increased for up to 40 min.

Finally, in hypocapnic hypoxia the situation is complicated by the threshold effect (Figure 3.3) shown by Nielsen & Smith (1952). The mechanism by which a threshold appears is very unclear. At first sight, CO_2 should have no effect on the horizontal limb of the dog-leg. Yet in subjects where the effect of isocapnic hypoxia was compared with that of spontaneously hypocapnic hypoxia, the degree of hypocapnic inhibition of the hypoxic response (which varied between individuals) was significantly correlated with the slope of the normoxic CO_2 response. In other words, a factor related to CO_2 sensitivity appeared to be operating in a region which should have been below the CO_2 threshold (Moore *et al.*, 1984).

In the Berkenbosch preparation of the anaesthetised cat with separately perfused central and peripheral chemoreceptors, no threshold for CO_2 was found for the central chemoreceptors, even when PCO_2 was decreased to 3 mmHg (0.4 kPa). It is most likely, therefore, that the apparently horizontal section of the dog-leg is composed of more than two drives (DeGoede *et al.*, 1981; Van Beek *et al.*, 1982; Berkenbosch *et al.*, 1984). The drive in man during hypocapnic hypoxia may include some component from the reticular system – perhaps the 'wakefulness' drive postulated by Fink (1963). The interpretation of the physiology of ventilatory control in hypocapnic hypoxia continues to provide the most difficult area in the overall response to CO_2.

3.10 The CO_2 response and exercise

During exercise, mean P_aCO_2 tends to remain constant despite large changes in CO_2 production. For this to occur, $\dot{V}_E$ must rise in direct proportion to V_{CO_2} as shown by eqn (3.2). Many workers have studied the response to inhaled CO_2 during exercise in the hope that it would shed some light on the way in which endogenous CO_2 might be controlling the hyperpnoea. The failure of mean P_aCO_2 to rise during exercise could, for example, be the result of a greatly increased sensitivity to CO_2. Despite considerable interest, no clear answer has emerged to the crucial question as to whether or not exercise alters the slope of the CO_2 response (see Flenley & Warren, 1983, for a recent review).

Using the classical method, Asmussen & Nielsen (1957) were amongst the first to compare CO_2 sensitivity at rest with that at various levels of exercise. The majority of their response curves had slopes of about the same magnitude, although in one subject the slope tended to increase with increasing work rate. They also noticed that during exercise the response curves tended to become flattened at the higher values of P_ACO_2.

Since then, the debate in general has been whether the slope is normal or increased in exercise. Clark & Godfrey (1969), using the rebreathing technique, actually found a significant decrease in the slope during steady-state exercise. Similar results were also obtained by Miyamura *et al.* (1976) with the rebreathing approach, but these authors considered rebreathing to be less reliable than the steady-state approach. Certainly, decreased CO_2 sensitivity with exercise seems to be found only by those adopting the rebreathing method. One possibility is that the increased CO_2 production during exercise will increase the rate of rise of PCO_2 in the rebreathing bag, thereby, altering the relationship between chemoreceptor and bag PCO_2. When bag size was adjusted so that the rate of rise of PCO_2 was the same during exercise as at rest, there was no difference in the slope of the response (Kelley *et al.*, 1982).

Leaving aside the special problems associated with rebreathing during exercise, there is still no consensus from those using the classical steady-state method; some workers find an increased slope and others report no change. Differences in technique may account for some of the inconsistencies: the subjects' posture, the exact method and concentrations used in the CO_2 administration, the means of measuring P_ACO_2 or P_aCO_2, and the type, duration and intensity of the exercise have all tended to vary from study to study. In particular, some workers have included the air-breathing point in their CO_2 responses while others have not. As the responses may flatten at the higher levels of P_ACO_2, the range over which the slope is measured is crucial and yet some workers have allowed P_ACO_2 to stray well over 60 mmHg (8.0 kPa). In these studies showing a decreased slope during rebreathing, values of about 100 mmHg (13.3 kPa) were not uncommon during exercise. Such values can hardly be considered as physiological; indeed, it could well be argued that the physiologically most interesting part of the response is the part closest to the normal control point – the very area that some workers have chosen to reject.

It is not possible to investigate the lower end of the response using rebreathing, and even using the classical method it is difficult to deliver a small CO_2 load with precision because the exact amount received by an exercising subject will depend on the $\dot{V}_E$ response to the exercise. In contrast, the constant inflow method allows small amounts of CO_2 to be delivered precisely regardless of the subject's $\dot{V}_E$, and P_ACO_2 will lie on a physiological hyperbola (Figure 3.1). Using this method, Cummin *et al.* (1986) have recently examined the response at rest and at various levels of exercise, concentrating on the region close to the control point. Their results show that at the lower end of the response there is a progressive increase in the slope with exercise and that, at higher levels of exercise, CO_2 sensitivity close to the control point may be very high indeed.

Poon & Greene (1985) approached the problem by maintaining P_aCO_2 constant at various levels of hypercapnia (up to 55 mmHg or 7.3 kPa) and then varying work rate under these isocapnic conditions. Their results, replotted in terms of the $\dot{V}_E$-P_aCO_2 relationship, show that the slope increases by a factor of 1.5–2.0 at a $\dot{V}_{CO_2}$ of 1.0 l·min^{-1} (about 50 W) and increases progressively with increasing work rate (the highest $\dot{V}_{CO_2}$ output studied was 1.5 l·min^{-1}). This type of response, together with the findings of Cummin *et al.* (1986) close to the control point, fits well with Poon's concept (1983) of a controller which balances the sum of the various drives to breathe with a propensity to minimise the associated respiratory work.

3.11 Applications in physiology, pharmacology and medicine

We shall not review the literature here but suggest that, in accordance with the principles outlined above, the reader may assess the importance of individual studies or reports by asking the following questions:

(a) Is the input variable appropriate (e.g $P_{ET}CO_2$ in exercise; effect of cerebral blood flow)?
(b) Is the output variable appropriate (total $\dot{V}$, $\dot{V}_A$, $P_{0.1}$)?
(c) What is the effect on slope?
(d) What is the effect on the PCO_2 intercept, or position, of the response line? (With the rebreathing technique, this cannot be assessed.)
(e) If changes are significant, what would be the effect on steady-state $\dot{V}_E$ and PCO_2 at rest and during exercise – see eqn (3.3)?
(f) Does it matter, in terms of control of breathing?
(g) Does it matter, in terms of CO_2 response as a defence mechanism?

3.12 **Further reading**

Cherniack, N. S. & Widdicombe, J. G. (eds) (1986). *Handbook of Physiology, Sect. 3, The Respiratory System*. American Physiological Society, Washington, D.C.

Hornbein, T. F. (ed.) (1981). *The Regulation of Breathing*, Vol. 17. Dekker, New York.

References

Anthonisen, N. R. & Dhingra, S. (1978). Ventilatory response to low levels of CO_2. *Respiration Physiology*, **32**, 335–44.

Asmussen, E. & Nielsen, M. (1957). Ventilatory response to CO_2 during work at normal and low oxygen tensions. *Acta Physiologica Scandinavica*, **39**, 27–35.

Berkenbosch, A., Van Beek, J. H. G. M., Olievier, C. N., DeGoede, J. & Quanjer, P. H. (1984). Central respiratory CO_2 sensitivity at extreme hypocapnia. *Respiration Physiology*, **55**, 95–102.

Bouverot, P., Flandrois, R., Puccinelli, R. & Dejours, P. (1965). Etude du role des chemorecepteurs arteriels dans la regulation de la respiration pulmonaire chez le chien eveille. *Archives Internationales de Pharmacodynamie* (*et de Therapie*), **157**, 253–71.

Britton, S. L., Lutherer, L. O. & Davies, D. G. (1979). Effect of cerebral extracellular fluid acidity on total and regional cerebral blood flow. *Journal of Applied Physiology*, **47**, 818–26.

Chambille, B., Guenard, H., Loncle, M. & Bargeton, D. (1975). Alveostat, an alveolar $PACO_2$ and PAO_2 control system. *Journal of Applied Physiology*, **39**, 837–42.

Chapman, R. W., Santiago, T. V. & Edelman, N. H. (1979). Effects of graded reduction of brain blood flow on ventilation in unanesthetised goats. *Journal of Applied Physiology*, **47**, 104–11.

Clark, T. J. H. & Godfrey, S. (1969). The effect of CO_2 on ventilation and breath-holding during exercise and while breathing through an added resistance. *Journal of Physiology*, **201**, 551–6.

Cummin, A. R. C., Alison, J., Jacobi, M. S., Iyawe, V. I. & Saunders, K. B. (1986). Ventilatory sensitivity to inhaled CO_2 around the control point during exercise. *Clinical Science*, **71**, 17–22.

Cunningham, D. J. C. (1974). Integrative aspects of the regulation of breathing: a personal view. In: *MTP International Review of Science*, Physiology, series 1, volume 2, *Respiratory Physiology*, pp. 303–69. University Park Press, Baltimore.

Daubenspeck, J. A. (1973). Frequency analysis of CO_2 regulation: afferent influences on tidal volume control. *Journal of Applied Physiology*, **35**, 662–72.

Davidson, A. C. & Cameron, I. R. (1985). Ventilatory control in normal man following five minutes exposure to hypoxia. *Respiration Physiology*, **60**, 227–36.

DeGoede, J., Berkenbosch, A., Olievier, C. N. & Quanjer, P. H. (1981). Ventilatory response to carbon dioxide and apnoeic thresholds. *Respiration Physiology*, **45**, 185–99.

DeGoede, J., Berkenbosch, A., Ward, D. S., Bellville, J. W. & Olievier, C. N. (1985). Comparison of chemoreflex gains obtained with two different methods in cats. *Journal of Applied Physiology*, **59**, 170–179.

Dejours, P. (1962). Chemoreflexes in breathing. *Physiological Reviews*, **42**, 335–58.

Dempsey, J. A. & Forster, H. V. (1982). Mediation of ventilatory adaptations. *Physiological Reviews*, **62**, 262–346.

Doblar, D. D., Min, B. G., Chapman, R. W., Harback, E. R., Welkowitz, W. & Edelman, N. H. (1979). Dynamic characteristics of cerebral blood flow response to sinusoidal hypoxia. *Journal of Applied Physiology*, **46**, 721–9.

Dubois, A. B., Britt, A. G. & Fenn, W. O. (1952). Alveolar CO_2 during the respiratory cycle. *Journal of Applied Physiology*, **4**, 535–48.

Eldridge, F. L., Kiley, J. P. & Millhorn, D. E. (1984). Respiratory effects of carbon dioxide-induced changes of medullary extracellular fluid pH in rats. *Journal of Physiology*, **355**, 177–89.

Eldridge, F. L., Millhorn, D. E. & Kiley, J. P. (1985). Antagonism by theophylline of respiratory inhibition induced by adenosine. *Journal of Applied Physiology*, **59**, 1428–33.

Fenn, W. O. & Craig, A. B. (1963). Effect of CO_2 on respiration using a new method of administering CO_2. *Journal of Applied Physiology*, **18**, 1023–4.

Feustel, P. J., Stafford, M. J., Allen, J. S. & Severinghaus, J. W. (1984). Ventrolateral medullary surface blood flow determined by hydrogen clearance. *Journal of Applied Physiology*, **56**, 150–4.

Fink, B. R., Hanks, E. C., Ngai, S. H. & Papper, E. M. (1963). Central regulation of respiration during anesthesia and wakefulness. *Annals of the New York Academy of Sciences*, **109**, 892–900.

Flenley, D. C. & Warren, P. M. (1983). Ventilatory responses to O_2 and CO_2 during exercise. *Annual Review of Physiology*, **45**, 415–26.

Folgering, H. T., Bernards, J. A., Biesta, J. H. & Smolders, F. (1974). Mathematical analysis of the response of lung ventilation to CO_2 in normoxia and hyperoxia. *Pflugers Archives*, **347**, 341–50.

Fordyce, W. E., Knuth, S. L. & Bartlett, D. (1984). Ventilatory responses to low levels of CO_2 inhalation in the cat. *Respiration Physiology*, **55**, 81–94.

Forster, H. V., Klein, J. P., Hamilton, L. H. & Kampine, J. M. (1982). Regulation of $PaCO_2$ and ventilation in humans inspiring low levels of CO_2. *Journal of Applied Physiology*, **52**, 287–94.

Gelb, A. F., Klein, E., Schiffman, P., Lugliani, R. & Aronstam. P. (1977). Ventilatory response and drive in acute and chronic obstructive pulmonary disease. *American Review of Respiratory Disease*, **116**, 9–16.

Haldane, J.S. & Priestley, J.G. (1905). The regulation of the lung-ventilation. *Journal of Physiology*, **32**, 225–66.

Hirsch, J.A. & Bishop, B. (1982). Human breathing patterns on mouthpiece or face mask during air, CO_2 or low O_2. *Journal of Applied Physiology*, **53**, 1281–90.

Honda, Y., Hata, N., Sakakibara, Y., Nishino, T. & Satomura, Y. (1981). Central hypoxic-hypercapnic interaction in mild hypoxia in man. *Pflugers Archives*, **391**, 289–95.

Hulsbosch, M.A.M., Binkhorst, R.A. & Folgering, H.T. (1982). Interaction of CO_2 and positive and negative exercise stimuli on the ventilation in man. *Pflugers Archives*, **394**, 16–20.

Jones, N.L., Robertson, D.G. & Kane, J.W. (1979). Difference between end-tidal and arterial PCO_2 in exercise. *Journal of Applied Physiology*, **47**, 954–60.

Kelley, M.A., Owens, G.R. & Fishman, A.P. (1982). Hypercapnic ventilation during exercise: Effects of exercise methods and inhalation techniques. *Respiration Physiology*, **50**, 75–85.

Linton, R.A.F., Poole-Wilson, P.A., Davies, R.J. & Cameron, I.R. (1973). A comparison of the ventilatory response to carbon dioxide by steady-state and rebreathing methods during metabolic acidosis and alkalosis. *Clinical Science*, **45**, 239–49.

Lloyd, B.B., Jukes, M.G.M. & Cunningham, D.J.C. (1958). The relation between alveolar oxygen pressure and the respiratory response to carbon dioxide in man. *Quarterly Journal of Experimental Physiology*, **43**, 214–27.

Lugliani, R., Whipp, B.J., Seard, C. & Wasserman, K. (1971). Effect of bilateral carotid-body resection on ventilatory control at rest and during exercise in man. *New England Journal of Medicine*, **285**, 1105–11.

Miller, J.P., Cunningham, D.J.C., Lloyd, B.B. & Young, J.M. (1974). The transient respiratory effects in man of sudden changes in alveolar CO_2 in hypoxia and in high oxygen. *Respiration Physiology*, **20**, 17–31.

Millhorn, D.E., Eldridge, F.L., Kiley, J.P. & Waldrop, T.G. (1984). Prolonged inhibition of respiration following acute hypoxia in glomectomized cats. *Respiration Physiology*, **57**, 331–40.

Miyamura, M., Yamashima, T. & Honda, Y. (1976). Ventilatory responses to CO_2 rebreathing at rest and during exercise in untrained subjects and athletes. *Japanese Journal of Physiology*, **26**, 245–54.

Moore, L.G., Huang, S.Y., McCullough, R.E., Sampson, J.B., Maher, J.T., Weil, J.V., Grover, R.F., Alexander, J.K. & Reeves, J.T. (1984). Variable inhibition by falling CO_2 of hypoxic ventilatory response in humans. *Journal of Applied Physiology*, **56**, 207–10.

Neubauer, J.A. & Edelman, N.H. (1984). Nonuniform brain blood flow response to hypoxia in unanesthetised cats. *Journal of Applied Physiology*, **57**, 1803–8.

Neubauer, J.A., Santiago, T.V., Posner, M.A. & Edelman, N.H. (1985). Ventral medullary pH and ventilatory responses to hyperperfusion and hypoxia. *Journal of Applied Physiology*, **58**, 1659–68.

Neubauer, J. A., Strumpf, D. A. & Edelman, N. H. (1983). Regional medullary blood flow during isocapnic hyperpnea in anaesthetized cats. *Journal of Applied Physiology*, **55**, 447–52.

Nielsen, M. & Smith, H. (1952). Studies on the regulation of respiration in acute hypoxia. *Acta Physiologica Scandinavica*, **24**, 293–313.

Olson, L. G., Hensley, M. J. & Saunders, N. A. (1982). Ventilatory responsiveness to hypercapnic hypoxia during dopamine infusion in humans. *American Review of Respiratory Disease*, **126**, 783–7.

Perez, W. & Tobin, M. J. (1985). Separation of factors responsible for change in breathing pattern induced by instrumentation. *Journal of Applied Physiology*, **59**, 1515–20.

Poon, C. S. (1983). Optimal control of ventilation in hypoxia, hypercapnia and exercise. In: *Modelling and Control of Breathing*, (Whipp, B. J. & Wiberg, D. M., eds.), pp. 189–96. Elsevier, New York.

Poon, C. S. & Greene, J. G. (1985). Control of exercise hyperpnea during hypercapnia in humans. *Journal of Applied Physiology*, **59**, 792–7.

Read, D. J. C. (1967). A clinical method for assessing the ventilatory response to carbon dioxide. *Australian Annals of Medicine*, **16**, 20–32.

Reischl, P., Stavert, D. M., Lewis, S. M., Murdock, L. C. & O'Louglin, B. J. (1980). End-tidal CO_2 response to low levels of inspired CO_2 in awake beagle dogs. *Journal of Applied Physiology*, **48**, 1077–82.

Reischl, P. & Stavert, D. M. (1982). Arterial CO_2 response to low levels of inspired CO_2 in awake beagle dogs. *Journal of Applied Physiology*, **52**, 672–6.

Riley, D. J., Santiago, T. V., Daniele, R. P., Schall, B. & Edelman, N. H. (1977). Blunted respiratory drive in congenital myopathy. *American Journal of Medicine*, **63**, 459–66.

Saunders, K. B., Bali, H. N. & Carson, E. R. (1980*a*). A breathing model of the respiratory system: the controlled system. *Journal of Theoretical Biology*, **84**, 135–61.

Saunders, K. B., Partridge, M. R. & Watson, A. C. (1980b). Inhalation of CO_2 by a constant-inflow technique at rest and during exercise. In: *Exercise Bioenergetics and Gas Exchange* (Cerretelli, P. & Whipp, B. J., eds.) pp. 223–234. Elsevier-North Holland, Amsterdam.

Severinghaus, J. W. (1976). Proposed standard determination of ventilatory responses to hypoxia and hypercapnia in man. *Chest*, **70**, 129–31.

Stoll, P. J. (1969). Respiratory system analysis based on sinusoidal variations of CO_2 in inspired air. *Journal of Applied Physiology*, **27**, 389–99.

Swanson, G. D. & Bellville, J. W. (1974). Hyperoxic-hypercapnic interaction in human respiratory control. *Journal of Applied Physiology*, **36**, 480–7.

Swanson, G. D. & Bellville, J. W. (1975). Step changes in end-tidal CO_2: methods and implications. *Journal of Applied Physiology*, **39**, 377–85.

Van Beek, J. H. G. M., Berkenbosch, A., DeGoede, J. & Olievier, C. N.

(1983). Influence of peripheral O_2 tension on the ventilatory response to CO_2 in cats. *Respiration Physiology*, **51**, 379–90.

Ward, S. A. & Whipp, B. J. (1980). Ventilatory control during exercise with increased external dead space. *Journal of Applied Physiology*, **48**, 225–31.

Weiskopf, R. B. & Gabel, R. A. (1975). Depression of ventilation during hypoxia in man. *Journal of Applied Physiology*, **39**, 911–5.

Weissman, C., Askanazi, J., Milic-Emili, J. & Kinney, J. M. (1984). Effect of respiratory apparatus on respiration. *Journal of Applied Physiology*, **57**, 475–80.

Whitelaw, W. A., Derenne, J. P. & Milic-Emili, J. (1975). Occlusion pressure as a measure of respiratory centre output in conscious man. *Respiration Physiology*, **23**, 181–99.

Wilson, D. A., Traystman, R. J. & Rapela, C. E. (1985). Transient analysis of the canine cerebrovascular response to carbon dioxide. *Circulation Research*, **56**, 596–605.

Yamamoto, W. S. (1980). Computer simulation of ventilatory control by both neural and humoral CO_2 signals. *American Journal of Physiology*, **238**, R28–R35.

4

Do oscillations in arterial CO_2 tension provide feed-forward control of ventilation?

B. A. Cross and S. J. G. Semple Departments of Medicine and Physiology, The Middlesex Hospital Medical School, London

4.1 **Introduction**

This chapter is concerned with the *experimental evidence* that **intra-breath oscillations** in arterial CO_2 tension (P_aCO_2) provide a signal for the **feed-forward control** of pulmonary ventilation ($\dot{V}_I$). The implication of such a control system is that $\dot{V}_I$ and the pulmonary exchange of CO_2 are appropriately matched to hold mean P_aCO_2 constant. This does not mean that the classical concepts and experiments describing the relationships between mean P_aCO_2 and $\dot{V}_I$ are invalid, nor that changes in mean P_aCO_2 do not change $\dot{V}_I$: there are certain special circumstances, such as during CO_2 inhalation and possibly in disease, when changes in mean P_aCO_2 may be important in controlling $\dot{V}_I$. However, during exercise of moderate intensity, a change in mean P_aCO_2 does not occur (see Chapter 5) and is therefore irrelevant. The theory of feed-forward control is dealt with by Cummin and Saunders in Chapter 3 and in an eminently readable publication by Saunders (1980) which is refreshingly free of mathematical and control theory jargon.

We shall thus describe how intra-breath P_aCO_2 oscillations could affect $\dot{V}_I$ without change in mean P_aCO_2, and the evidence that this is so. Where possible we will relate the oscillations directly to $\dot{V}_I$, but in many instances the correlation will be with carotid chemoreceptor discharge and hence the link with $\dot{V}_I$ is indirect and not always certain.

4.2 Measurement of pH as a reflection of arterial CO_2 tension

The intra-breath oscillations in arterial pH (pH_a) are technically much easier to record and measure than are those in P_aCO_2. In most of the experimental work we shall quote, pH_a oscillations have been measured on the assumption that they reflect corresponding oscillations in P_aCO_2. The justification for this is that the amplitude of the pH_a oscillations is compatible with their arising from fluctuations in alveolar PCO_2 (P_ACO_2) and that modifications in the contour of these fluctuations by various means are reflected in the pH_a oscillations (Band *et al.*, 1969*b*). In addition, simultaneous measurements of P_aCO_2 and pH_a oscillations with appropriate electrodes have shown that they can be solely accounted for by changes in P_aCO_2 (Plaas-Link, 1981).

Oscillations in pHa have been recorded in man (Band & Semple, 1966), dog (Cross *et al.*, 1979*a* and *b*) and cat (Band *et al.*, 1969*a*). Their amplitude at rest varies directly with tidal volume (V_T) and inversely with breathing frequency (f); the latter having the dominant effect. In the cat, oscillations can still be recorded at rates in excess of $35\,min^{-1}$, but it is currently uncertain whether they are present at such high rates in man.

How can an oscillating chemical signal produce a different stimulus to breathing from that induced by a constant stimulus? After all, the rise in PCO_2 and the fall in PO_2 during expiration should be counteracted by the fall in PCO_2 and rise in PO_2 during inspiration. This is only true, however, if the respiratory response to a chemical stimulus is constant in amplitude and direction throughout the respiratory cycle. In fact, this is not so: the response to a given stimulus is greater in late than early inspiration, and is absent or opposite in direction during expiration (Black & Torrance, 1967; Band *et al.*, 1970; Eldridge, 1976; Nye *et al.*, 1981).

Figure 4.1 shows a record of V_T and the carotid artery pH oscillation in an anaesthetised cat. Injections of saline equilibrated with 100% CO_2 given via a catheter in the root of the aorta produced small acid deflections in pH similar in magnitude to the amplitude of the naturally occurring oscillations; although a respiratory effect only occurred when the injections were correctly timed in the respiratory cycle. In contrast, correctly

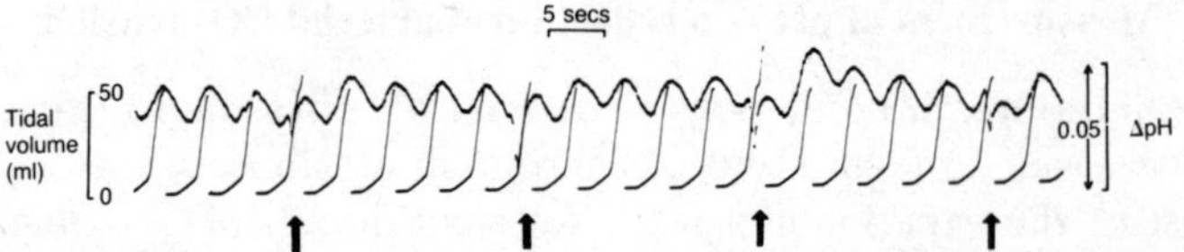

Fig. 4.1 Carotid artery pH (upper trace: alkaline changes upward) and tidal volume (lower trace) responses in an anaesthetized cat to four consecutive injections (at arrows) of saline (0.3 ml) equilibrated with 100% CO_2 administered via a catheter in the root of the aorta. Injections 1 and 3 caused V_T to increase; however, injection 2 was timed too early and injection 4 too late in inspiration to produce an effect.

timed injections of non-gaseous acids (e.g. lactic acid and hydrochloric acid) were without effect. This difference in respiratory effect between gaseous and non-gaseous acids is due to the slow dehydration of carbonic acid in plasma. When hydrochloric acid is injected into the plasma, the following reactions take place:

$$HCl + NaHCO_3 \rightarrow NaCl + H_2CO_3 \tag{4.1}$$

$$H_2CO_3 \rightleftharpoons H_2O + CO_2 \tag{4.2}$$

Reaction (4.1) is virtually instantaneous but reaction (4.2) is slow in plasma where carbonic anhydrase is absent, so that little CO_2 is formed in the short circulation time between the root of the aorta (site of injection) and the carotid body (~2 s). This specific respiratory effect of CO_2 can be accounted for on the basis that it is freely diffusible across the tissues separating plasma from the carotid chemoreceptors, whereas H^+ ions are not. The experimental evidence for this assertion is that when a non-gaseous acid is injected *together* with carbonic anhydrase, the chemoreceptors are stimulated whereas acid alone has no such effect (Band *et al.*, 1978). Carbonic anhydrase is present in the carotid body, so that changes in PCO_2 will lead to corresponding alterations in $[H^+]$; changes in $[H^+]$ within the extravascular environment of the chemoreceptors may still therefore be the ultimate stimulus to those receptors.

4.3 **The timing effect**

The effect of timing of a chemical stimulus on $\dot{V}_I$ is illustrated in two schematic representations of V_T and the P_aCO_2 oscillations

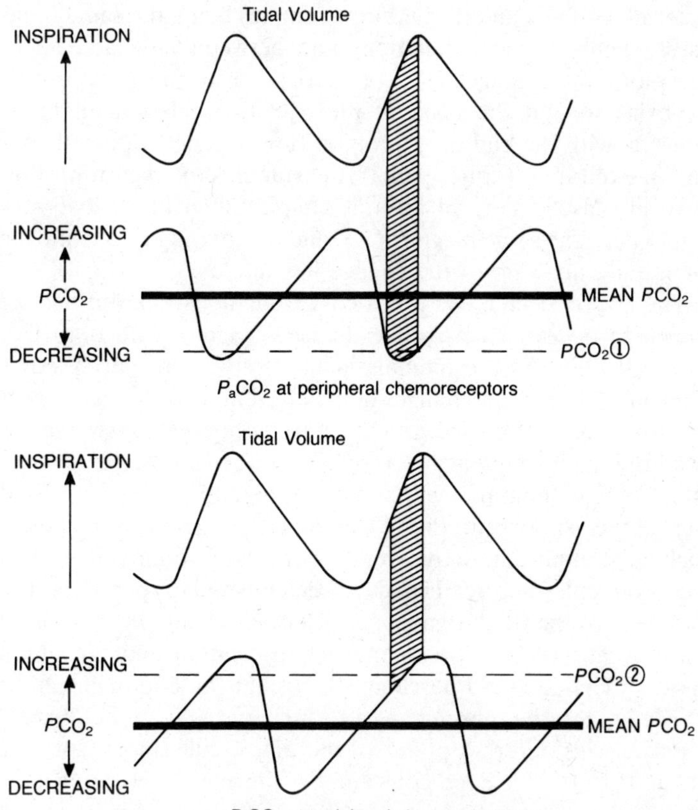

Fig. 4.2 Schematic representation of two possible phase relationships between the respiratory cycle (upper traces) and P_aCO_2 oscillations (lower traces). Humoral signals received during the last half of inspiration (hatched area) have the most potent effect on $\dot{V}_I$: in the upper panel, this region coincides with the trough of the P_aCO_2 oscillation, PCO_2 (1) and, in the lower panel, with the peak of the oscillation, PCO_2 (2). Mean P_aCO_2 (bold horizontal lines) is identical in both cases.

(Figure 4.2): in the upper panel, the P_aCO_2 oscillation has been drawn so that its trough coincides with the end of inspiration while, in the lower panel, its peak coincides with the end of inspiration. Since the end of inspiration is the most sensitive part of the respiratory cycle, the stimulus to breathing could be different in the two situations, despite the mean P_aCO_2 (as determined from an arterial blood sample) being the same in both cases. Thus, if the circulation time between lung and chemoreceptors now changes (e.g. at exercise onset or on exposure to hypoxia) so that the peak of the P_aCO_2 oscillation might now coincide with the end of inspiration (lower panel) rather than the end of expiration (upper panel), the stimulus to respiration would have increased. Yet, an arterial sample taken in the two states would have the same *mean* P_aCO_2 and the investigator would have been quite unaware of the change in stimulus.

The above mechanism is not easy to demonstrate but has been shown to operate in the anaesthetised, vagotomised dog (Cross *et al.*, 1979*a*). As the animals in this study were paralysed and artificially ventilated, changes in the efferent drive to breathe were assessed from the 'integrated' phrenic nerve discharge, the amplitude and frequency of which have been shown to reflect V_T and f of the spontaneously-breathing animal accurately. At the start of the experiment, the ventilator was triggered by the onset of each burst of phrenic activity to deliver a fixed volume of air. Once measurements had been made, a delay was interposed between the onset of the discharge and the delivery of air. In this way the phase relationship between the pH_a oscillation and the phrenic nerve discharge could be changed, so that the end of inspiration (the peak of the phrenic nerve discharge) could be made to coincide with different points of the pH_a oscillation (Figure 4.2). Mean P_aCO_2 was kept constant by altering the volume of air delivered by the ventilator, so that any alteration in phrenic nerve output was solely determined by changes in the phase relationship between pHa and the respiratory cycle. The main effect of alterations in this phase relationship was on expiratory time (T_E), where changes of up to 30% were produced; this effect was abolished by peripheral chemoreceptor denervation.

4.4 **Phase relationship and ventilatory control**

In the spontaneously breathing animal, such alterations in the phase relationship might be brought about by changes in circulation time between lung and peripheral chemoreceptors and/or by changes in f set by the bulbopontine rhythm generator. The precise role of the phase relationship between respiratory and pH_a

cycles in ventilatory control in man remains to be determined; it has been shown, however, that changes in this relationship do affect $\dot{V}_I$ in man during moderate hypoxia (Cunningham *et al.*, 1983*a* and *b*). From the results of the study on dogs described above (Cross *et al.*, 1979*a*) as well as those on spontaneously breathing animals, it can be expected that changes in $\dot{V}_I$ of about 17% could be produced by alterations solely in the phase relationship (Cross *et al.*, 1979*b*). The most likely role for this control mechanism is in the fine tuning of breathing at rest and in sleep, especially when f is low and V_T is large; a condition which would produce pH_a oscillations of large amplitude. So far, the experimental evidence is that changes in the phase relationship play no part in the $\dot{V}_I$ response to exercise (Petersen *et al.*, 1978; Cross *et al.*, 1982*b*).

Whilst alterations in the phase relationship between the respiratory and pH_a cycles may influence breathing, these alterations do not provide a mechanism for the matching of $\dot{V}_I$ to CO_2 output ($\dot{V}_{CO_2}$) such that P_aCO_2 remains constant when metabolic CO_2 production or the CO_2 delivery to the lungs is altered by a change in cardiac output and hence venous return. A potential humoral signal for this matching has been proposed on theoretical grounds and from mathematical modelling of the ventilatory control system (Saunders, 1980). The potential signal is the slope of the upstroke of the P_aCO_2 oscillation; this can be understood intuitively. During expiration, when the upstroke of the oscillation is generated in the lung, there is no fresh air entering gas-exchange areas; the upstroke will thus be solely dependent on the pulmonary CO_2 flux from mixed venous blood into the alveoli which will in turn reflect metabolic CO_2 production and cardiac output. Changes in V_T and f (and thus in $\dot{V}_I$) will affect mean P_aCO_2 as well as the downstroke of the oscillation, but will not change the slope of the upstroke (although f will affect its duration) (Figure 4.3).

Theoretical analysis of the factors determining the P_aCO_2 oscillations predicts that the slope of the upstroke will be linearly related to pulmonary CO_2 flux and, for the reasons given in the preceding paragraphs, will be independent of $\dot{V}_I$. Direct experimental evidence that this is so has been provided from experiments in the anaesthetized cat (Cross *et al.*, 1981) using a

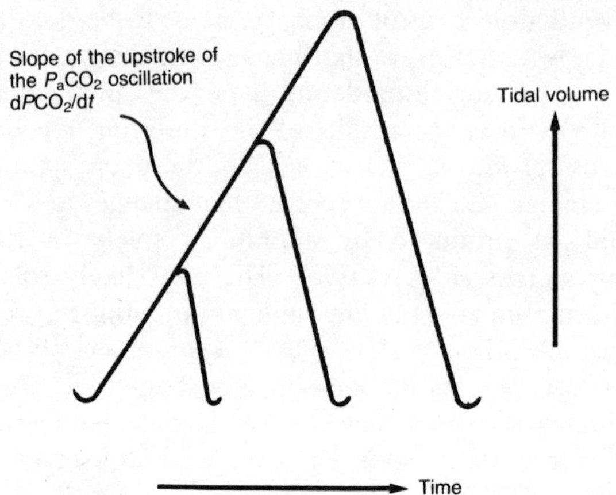

Fig. 4.3 Schematic representation of the P_aCO_2 oscillation to illustrate how the slope of the upstroke ($dPCO_2/dt$) can be unaffected by variations in tidal volume and breath duration. Note, however, that the duration of the upstroke increases as the duration of the breath becomes longer.

technique first described in cats by Nye & Marsh (1982): $\dot{V}_{CO_2}$ was increased by passing gas of high CO_2 content through the intestines and was reduced by perfusing them with Tris buffer (tris-hydroxymethylaminomethane) which combines chemically with CO_2. Figure 4.4 shows the results of such an experiment where it can be seen that $\dot{V}_{CO_2}$ is linearly related to the maximum rate of change of the upstroke of the PCO_2 oscillation ($dPCO_2/dt \uparrow max$) (*the maximum* rate of change has been chosen because it is determined by the linear part of the upstroke and is a convenient and satisfactory index for the slope of the whole upstroke).

Changes in $dPCO_2/dt \uparrow$ max provide a potential chemical signal to $\dot{V}_I$ during exercise which would ensure that $\dot{V}_I$ was matched to pulmonary CO_2 flux without change in mean P_aCO_2. At exercise onset (i.e. for the initial 10–15 s), the increased CO_2 flux would be determined by the immediate increase in the volume of blood reaching the lung rather than by a change in its CO_2 content, as there would not have been enough time for blood to have travelled from the exercising limbs to the lung; as exercise proceeds, the mixed venous CO_2 content would rise, leading to a further increase in CO_2 flux. If, as suggested by Wasserman *et al.* (1981), $\dot{V}_I$ during exercise is coupled to pulmonary CO_2 delivery, then the

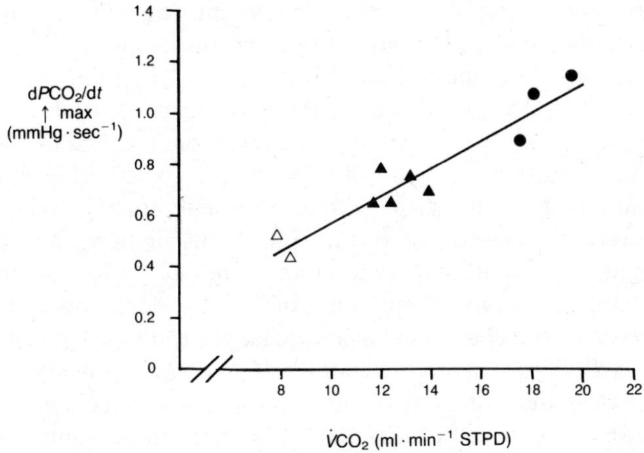

Fig. 4.4 Linear association between the maximum rate of change of the upstroke of the P_aCO_2 oscillation ($dPCO_2/dt \uparrow$ max) and CO_2 output ($\dot{V}_{CO_2}$) in an anaesthetized cat under control conditions (▲), with $\dot{V}_{CO_2}$ increased by passing high-CO_2 gas through the small intestine (●) and reduced by perfusing intestine with Tris buffer (△).

slope of the upstroke of the PCO_2 oscillation may be the humoral signal responsible for the coupling. As the signal is a slope and not an absolute value, then a transducer must be found in the arterial circulation which responds to a rate of PCO_2 change; the likely transducer is the carotid body.

4.5 **The role of the carotid body**

Carotid body chemoreceptor activity, recorded from carotid sinus nerve afferents, exhibits fluctuations which have the same frequency as the respiratory cycle. This observation, first made by Hornbein *et al.* in 1961, has since been repeated by a number of workers. Based on the response characteristics of the chemoreceptors to changes in P_aCO_2 and P_aO_2 (typically imposed as step or oscillatory functions), the fluctuations in chemoreceptors discharge have been attributed primarily to the intra-breath P_aCO_2 oscillations. However, the relationship between chemoreceptor discharge and the P_aCO_2 oscillations is not one of simple proportion. The fluctuations in discharge, recorded under normoxic conditions from few or single fibre carotid sinus nerve preparations, are large relative to the mean discharge (Biscoe & Purves, 1967; Goodman *et al.*, 1974; Band *et al.*, 1978), whereas the predicted P_aCO_2 oscillations are by comparison small relative to the mean P_aCO_2. Either the chemoreceptors respond to P_aCO_2 with high gain and high threshold or with a dynamic sensitivity. Evidence that there is a large rate-of-change component in the chemoreceptor response to the P_aCO_2 oscillations has been obtained by comparing the amplitude of the *fluctuating* discharge associated with a given amplitude of P_aCO_2 oscillation with the amplitude of the change in *mean* discharge produced by a change in mean P_aCO_2 of similar magnitude (Cross *et al.*, 1984*a*).

To assess the potential of these receptors to mediate the $\dot{V}_I$ response to changes in pulmonary CO_2 flux, these studies were extended to determine the sensitivity of carotid chemoreceptors in the cat to changes in the rate of rise of the P_aCO_2 oscillation (Cross *et al.*, 1984*b*). The rate of rise of the oscillation was increased by passing gas of high CO_2 content through the small intestines of anaesthetised, paralysed cats which were ventilated at constant frequency (this ensured a constant P_aCO_2 cycle duration and facilitated bin-averaging of the nerve discharge associated with the oscillations). Chemoreceptor activity recorded from few or many fibre carotid sinus nerve preparations was averaged over a minimum of 20 respiratory cycles during the control periods before and after CO_2 loading and also at least 10 min after the start of CO_2 loading. By increasing the volume delivered by the ventilator during CO_2 loading, changes in mean P_aCO_2 were minimised. The effect of changes in the rate of rise of the P_aCO_2 oscillation could therefore be assessed in the absence of changes in mean P_aCO_2. Based on the earlier observation that the amplitude of the fluctuation in discharge was a function of the rate of change of the P_aCO_2 oscillation, it was hypothesised that the amplitude of the fluctuation in chemoreceptor discharge should increase when the rate of rise of the oscillation is increased. The amplitude of the fluctuation in discharge *did* increase during CO_2 loading, but only when increases in P_aO_2 associated with increasing the stroke volume of the ventilator were prevented by simultaneously adjusting the inspired PO_2 (Figure 4.5). A transducer responsive to the rate of rise of the PCO_2 oscillation therefore exists within

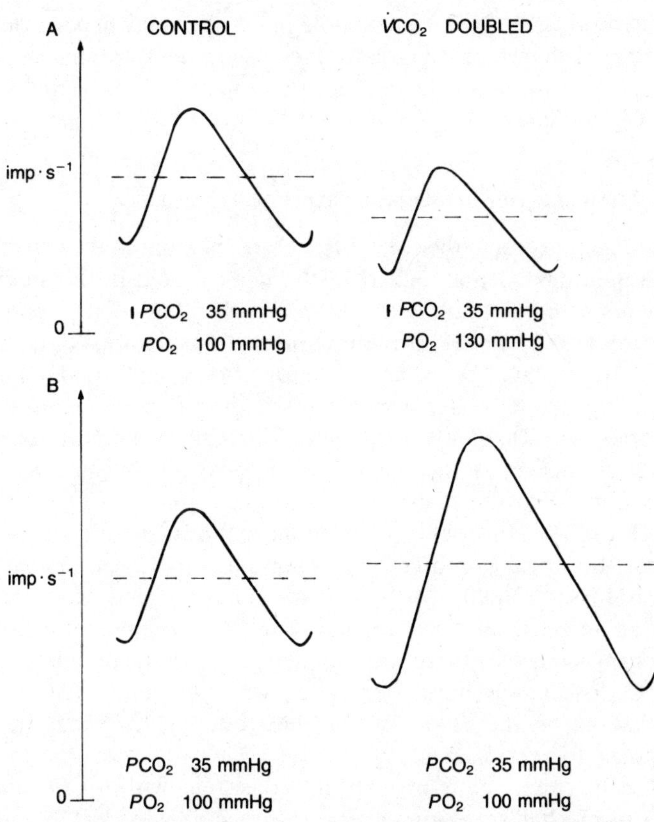

Fig. 4.5 Schematic representation of the effect on fluctuating carotid chemoreceptor discharge (measured in impulses per second, $imp \cdot s^{-1}$) of increasing CO_2 output ($\dot{V}_{CO_2}$), with mean P_aCO_2 constant. In response to a doubling of $\dot{V}_{CO_2}$, both the amplitude of the fluctuation and the mean level of discharge (dashed line) are increased when arterial PO_2 is maintained constant at 100 mmHg or 13.3 kPa (B), but are reduced if PO_2 rises (130 mmHg or 17.3 kPa) (A).

the carotid body. However, its role in exercise may depend on the associated change in P_aO_2, since increases in PO_2 as small as 10% were found to modulate the sensitivity to this component of the P_aCO_2 oscillation.

4.6 A possible role in mediating exercise hyperpnoea

Although interest in the role of P_aCO_2 oscillations in the control of breathing has been extended to the clinical field in the study of patients with heart failure (Band & Semple, 1966) and respiratory disease (Cochrane *et al.*, 1981) most considerations of these oscillations have been directed towards a proposed role in mediating exercise hyperpnoea. In addition to the neurogenic theories (see Chapter 5 for detailed discussion), humoral control of $\dot{V}_I$ during exercise can be divided into two possible mechanisms. The first is that there are changes in mean pH_a, P_aCO_2 or P_aO_2 which can account for the $\dot{V}_I$ response. Whilst these changes are small, their effect on breathing is amplified by (*a*) an increase in respiratory sensitivity of the control system during exercise and (*b*) an increase in body temperature. The second of the two mechanisms is that there are changes in the characteristics of the P_aCO_2 oscillation during exercise, with the amplitude of the oscillation or the slope of the upstroke determining the $\dot{V}_I$ response to exercise.

Recent experiments in man are consistent with a CO_2-linked control mechanism during exercise (cf., *a* above). For example, electrically induced exercise (E_{el}) can be produced in conscious man by surface-electrode stimulation of the quadriceps and hamstring muscles to produce a rhythmic pushing movement against a spring load. This technique has been found to produce no pain or discomfort (Adams *et al.*, 1984). E_{el} can be matched to voluntary exercise (E_v) by subjects copying a tension curve recorded during E_{el} which is displayed on an oscilloscope. The $\dot{V}_I$ response was the same in the two types of experiment, except for one interesting difference at the start of exercise: T_E of the first breath in which exercise was started was shortened in E_v and not E_{el} (Figure 4.6), causing $\dot{V}_I$ also to increase (when this is computed breath-by-breath). Thus, when exercise is started by a command from the investigator during expiration, the command

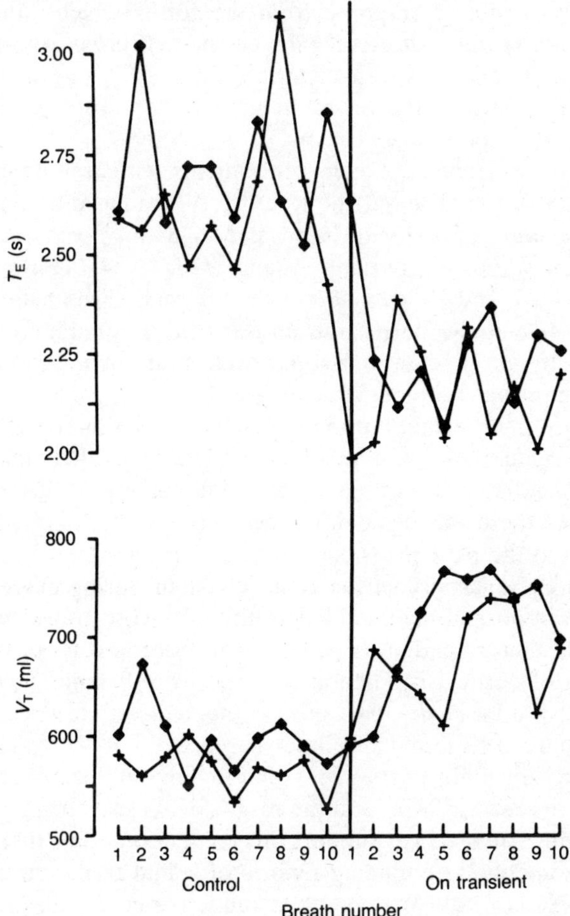

Fig. 4.6 Mean breath-by-breath responses of expiratory duration (T_E) and ventilation ($\dot{V}_T$) to on-transients of volitionally-induced exercise (E_v: +; $n = 23$) and electrically-induced exercise (E_{el}: ◆; $n = 31$) in man. The vertical line indicates the breath (during expiration) in which exercise began. Analysis of variance shows that the first significant shortening of T_E occurs on breath 1 for E_v and breath 2 for E_{el}; the first significant increase for $\dot{V}_T$ occurred on breath 2 for E_v and breath 3 for E_{el}.

probably triggers a response from the cortex which initiates an inspiration thereby shortening T_E on the first breath of exercise. However, in all other respects, the results of E_{el} suggest that the voluntary control of exercise in man is not necessary for the ventilatory response.

Electrically-induced exercise in patients with traumatic spinal cord transection at about the level of T6 produced a ventilatory response which, when expressed as $\Delta\dot{V}_I/\Delta\dot{V}_{CO_2}$, was not significantly different from normal (Adams *et al.*, 1984). However, the rises in $\dot{V}_{CO_2}$ and $\dot{V}_I$ were slower than normal in the patients and the increase in $\dot{V}_I$ during the on-transient was achieved almost entirely by an increase in V_T; in normals, an increase in f was a more important component (Figure 4.7). The reason for this difference is uncertain but may be due to loss a motor control of the lower intercostals, abdominal muscles and other muscles of posture leading to a different pattern of breathing. If this were the case, then there may be no difference in the control of breathing in exercise in the patients as compared with the normal subjects.

From these experiments on the effect of electrically induced exercise in normal man and in patients with cord transection, we conclude that a ventilatory response to exercise can occur in the absence of cortical irradiation to a sub-hypothalamic locomotor centre (Eldridge *et al.*, 1981) or to pontomedullary centres (Krogh & Lindhard, 1913), and also in the absence of normal signals from the exercising limbs (Kao, 1963). Our findings in the anaesthetised dog (Cross *et al.*, 1982*a*) and the results of Weissman *et al.* (1980) in the anaesthetised cat support this contention. (For discussions of the sometimes conflicting reports of spinal transection on $\dot{V}_I$ during exercise, see Whipp, 1981, and Cross *et al.*, 1982*a*.)

The matching of $\dot{V}_I$ to $\dot{V}_{CO_2}$ thus appears to be a consistent feature of the ventilatory response to exercise in these and other experiments, both for man and animals. Consequently, there is no consistent or significant change in mean P_aCO_2. This cannot be explained on the basis of classical chemoreception and it is likely that there is an, as yet, undefined humoral stimulus. This stimulus could be the slope of the upstroke of the P_aCO_2 oscillation; the peripheral chemoreceptors acting as the transducer. The signal is highly appropriate for the known $\dot{V}_I$ response to exercise, in that the slope of the upstroke is linearly related to $\dot{V}_{CO_2}$. Changes in

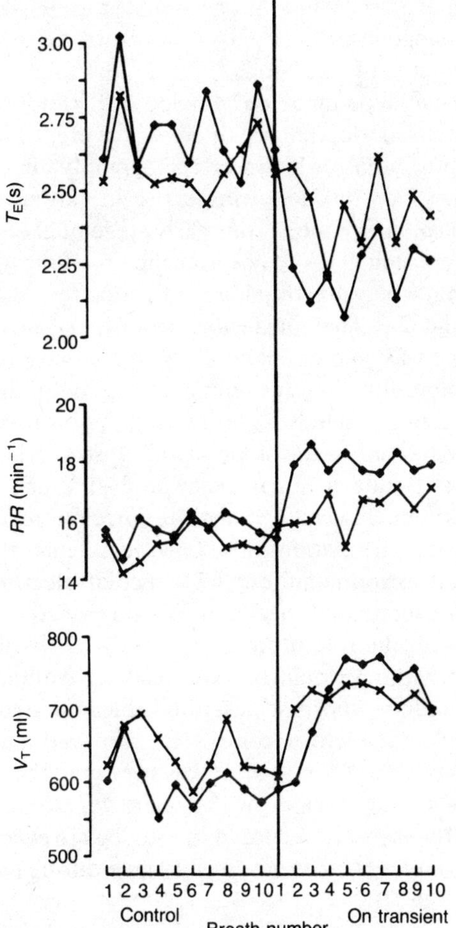

Fig. 4.7 Mean breath-by-breath responses of expiratory duration (T_E), respiratory rate (*RR*) and tidal volume (V_T) to on-transients of electrically-induced exercise for patients with spinal transection (× ; $n = 32$) and normals (◆; $n = 31$). The vertical line indicates the breath (during expiration) in which exercise began. In the patients, T_E changes more slowly, the rise in *RR* is slower and smaller, and V_T changes more rapidly than in normals.

the slope on exercise could thus account for the $\dot{V}_I$-$\dot{V}_{CO_2}$ matching without a change in mean P_aCO_2.

Measurements of the slope of the upstroke of the P_aCO_2 oscillation have been made during electrically induced exercise in the anaesthetised dog. Slope increases were observed by the second or third breath which were presumably due to an increase in pulmonary CO_2 flux following a rise in cardiac output (there would not have been time, at this early stage of exercise, for blood from the exercising limbs to have reached the lungs). Correlations were then made between the slope of the upstroke and the changes in $\dot{V}_I$, V_T and T_E. The conclusions from these correlations were that the slope was a potential humoral signal in exercise and could totally account for the shortening in T_E both during the on-transient and in the steady state. During the on-transient, $\dot{V}_I$ was also linearly related to the slope of the upstroke but there was a late rise in $\dot{V}_I$ (due to an increase in V_T) which could not be accounted for in this way. Statistical correlations do not necessarily imply causal relationships, however. Thus, the role of the slope of the upstroke of the P_aCO_2 oscillation in the control of breathing in exercise still needs to be established.

A chapter on the role of intra-breath P_aCO_2 oscillations in the control of breathing would be sadly lacking without a tribute to Yamamoto (1960) who first described the potential role of such oscillations in ventilatory control at rest and during exercise (Yamamoto & Edwards, 1960). It was twenty years before the first publications of the changes in the characteristics of these oscillations on exercise were recorded in the dog (Brewer *et al.*, 1979). Since then, similar records have been made during exercise in man (Band *et al.*, 1980).

4.7 **Further reading**

Cunningham, D. J. (1974). The control system regulating breathing in man. *Quarterly Reviews of Biophysics*, **6**(4), 443–83.

Semple, S. J. G. (1984). The role of oscillations in arterial CO_2 tension in the chemical control of breathing at rest and on exercise. *Clinical Science*, **66**, 639–42.

Symposium on ventilatory control during exercise (1979). *Medicine and Science in Sport*, **11**(2), 190–226.

Wasserman, K., Whipp, B. J. & Davis, J. A. (1981). Respiratory physiology of exercise. Metabolism, gas exchange and ventilatory control. In: *International Review of Physiology, Respiratory Physiology III*, (Widdicombe, J. G., ed.), pp. 149–211. University Park Press, Baltimore.

References

Adams, L., Frankel, H., Garlick, J., Guz, A., Murphy, K. & Semple, S. J. G. (1984). The role of the spinal cord transmission in the ventilatory response to exercise in man. *Journal of Physiology*, **355**, 85–97.

Adams, L., Garlick, J., Guz, A., Murphy, K. & Semple, S. J. G. (1984). Is the voluntary control of exercise in man necessary for the ventilatory response? *Journal of Physiology*, **355**, 71–83.

Adams, L., Guz, A., Innes, J. A. & Murphy, K. (1985*a*). The circulatory response to voluntary and electrically induced exercise in man. *Journal of Physiology*, **365**, 99P.

Adams, L., Guz, A., Innes, J. A. & Murphy, K. (1985*b*). Dynamics of the early ventilatory responses to voluntary and electrically induced exercise in man. *Journal of Physiology*, **369**, 142P.

Band, D. M. & Semple, S. J. G. (1966). In: *Breathlessness*, (Howell, J. B. L. & Campbell, E. J. M., eds.) p. 124. Blackwell, Oxford.

Band, D. M., Cameron, I. R. & Semple, S. J. G. (1969*a*). Oscillations in arterial pH with breathing in the cat. *Journal of Applied Physiology*, **26**, 261–7.

Band, D. M., Cameron, I. R. & Semple, S. J. G. (1969*b*). Effect of different methods of CO_2 administration on oscillations of arterial pH in the cat. *Journal of Applied Physiology*, **26**, 268–73.

Band, D. M., Cameron, I. R. & Semple, S. J. G. (1970). The effect on respiration of abrupt changes in carotid artery pH and P_{CO2} in the cat. *Journal of Applied Physiology*, **211**, 479–94.

Band, D. M., McClelland, M., Phillips, D., Saunders, K. & Wolff, C. B. (1978). Sensitivity of the carotid body to within breath changes in arterial P_{CO2}. Sensitivity of the carotid body to within breath changes in arterial P_{CO2}. *Journal of Applied Physiology*, **45**, 768–77.

Band, D. M., Wolff, C. B., Ward, J., Cochrane, G. M. & Prior, J. (1980). Respiratory oscillations in arterial carbon dioxide tension as a control signal in exercise. *Nature*, **283**, 84–5.

Biscoe, T. J. & Purves, M. J. (1967). Observations on the rhythmic variation in the cat carotid body chemoreceptor activity which has the same period as respiration. *Journal of Physiology*, **190**, 389–412.

Black, A. M. S., Goodman, N. W., Nail, B. S., Rao, P. S. & Torrance, R. W. (1973). The significance of the timing of chemoreceptor discharge impulses for their effect upon respiration. *Acta Neurobiologiae Experimentalis*, **33**, 139–47.

Black, A. M. S. & Torrance, R. W. (1967). Chemoreceptor effects in the respiratory cycle. *Journal of Physiology*, **189**, 59–60P.

Brewer, A., Cross, B. A., Davey, A., Guz, A., Jones P. W., Katona, P., Maclean, M. Murphy, K., Semple, S. J. G., Solomon, M. A. & Stidwill, R. P. (1979). Effect of electrically induced exercise in anaesthetised dogs on ventilation and arterial pH. *Journal of Physiology*, **298**, 49–50P.

Cochrane, G. M., Prior, J. G. & Wolff, C. B. (1981). Respiratory arterial pH and P_{CO2} oscillations in patients with obstructive airways disease. *Clinical Science*, **61**, 693–702.

Cross, B. A., Davey, A., Guz, A., Katona, P. G., Maclean, M., Murphy, K., Semple, S. J. G. & Stidwill, R. P. (1982*a*). The role of spinal cord transmission in the ventilatory response to electrically induced exercise in the anaesthetised dog. *Journal of Physiology*, **329**, 37–55.

Cross, B. A., Davey, A., Guz, A., Katona, P. G., Maclean, M., Murphy, K., Semple, S. J. G. & Stidwill, R. P. (1982*b*). The pH oscillation in arterial blood during exercise; a potential signal for the ventilatory response in the dog. *Journal of Physiology*, **329**, 57–73.

Cross, B. A., Grant, B. J. B., Guz, A., Jones, P. W., Semple, S. J. G. & Stidwill, R. P. (1979*a*). Dependence of phrenic motorneurone output on the oscillatory component of arterial blood gas composition. *Journal of Physiology*, **290**, 163–84.

Cross, B. A., Grant, B. J. B., Guz, A., Jones, P. W., Semple, S. J. G. & Stidwill, R. P. (1979*b*). An assessment of the effect of the oscillatory component of arterial blood gas composition on pulmonary ventilation. In: *Central Nervous Control Mechanisms in Breathing*, (Von Euler, C. & Lagercrantz, H., eds.), pp. 91–4. Pergamon, New York.

Cross, B. A., Jones, P. W., Leaver, K. D., Semple, S. J. G. & Stidwill, R. P. (1981). The relationship between CO_2 output, pulmonary ventilation and the rate of change of arterial pH of the downstroke of the oscillation in the cat. *Journal of Physiology*, **320**, 100–101P.

Cross, B. A., Leaver, K. D., Semple, S. J. G. & Stidwill, R. P. (1984*a*). Response of carotid body chemoreceptor discharge to small changes in $PaCO_2$ in the cat. *Journal of Physiology*, **353**, 131P.

Cross, B. A., Leaver, K. D., Semple, S. J. G. & Stidwill, R. P. (1984*b*). Response of carotid chemoreceptor discharge to alterations in the slope of the arterial pH oscillation in the cat. *Journal of Physiology*, **357**, 90P.

Cunningham, D. J. C., Howson, M. G., Metias, E. F. & Petersen, E. S. (1983*a*). Patterns of reflex responses to dynamic stimulation of the human respiratory system. In: *Central Neurone Environment and the Control Systems of Breathing and Circulation* (Schlaefke, M. E., Koepchen, H. P. & See, W. R., eds.), pp. 116–23. Springer-Verlag, Berlin.

Cunningham, D. J. C., Howson, M. G., Metias, E. F. & Peterson, E. S.

(1983*b*). Reflex responses to dynamic stimulation of the human respiratory system. *Journal of Physiology*, **345**, 173P.

Eldridge, F. L. (1972). The importance of timing on the respiratory effects of intermittent carotid body chemoreceptor stimulation. *Journal of Physiology*, **222**, 319–33.

Eldridge, F. L. (1976). Expiratory effects of brief carotid sinus nerve and carotid body stimulation. *Respiration Physiology*, **26**, 395–410.

Eldridge, E. L., Milhorn, D. E. & Waldrop, T. G. (1981). Exercise hyperpnea and locomotion: Parallel activation from the hypothalamus. *Science*, **221**, 844–6.

Goodman, N. W., Nail, B. S. & Torrance, R. W. (1974). Oscillations in the discharge of single carotid chemoreceptor fibres in the cat. *Respiration Physiology*, **20**, 251–63.

Hornbein, T. F., Griffo, Z. J. & Roos, A. (1961). Quantitation of chemoreceptor activity: interrelation of hypoxia and hypercapnia. *Journal of Neurophysiology*, **24**, 561–8.

Kao, F. F. (1963). An experimental study of the pathways involved in exercise hyperpnoea employing cross circulation techniques. In: *The Regulation of Human Respiration* (Cunningham, D. J. C. & Lloyd, B. B., eds.), pp. 461–502. Blackwell, Oxford.

Krogh, A. & Lindhard, J. (1913). The regulation of respiration and circulation during the initial stages of muscular work. *Journal of Physiology*, **47**, 112–36.

Nye, P. C. G., Hanson, M. A. & Torrance, R. W. (1981). The effect on breathing of abruptly stopping carotid body discharge. *Respiration Physiology*, **46**, 309–26.

Nye, P. C. G. & Marsh, J. (1982). Ventilation and carotid chemoreceptor discharge during CO_2 loading via the gut. *Respiration Physiology*, **50**, 335–50.

Petersen, E. S., Whipp, B. J., Drysdale, D. B. & Cunningham, D. J. C. (1978). The relation between arterial blood gas oscillations in the carotid region and the phase of the respiratory cycle during exercise in man: Testing a model. In: *Regulation of Respiration during Sleep and Anesthesia* (Fitzgerald, R., Gautier, H. & Lahiri, S., eds.), pp. 335–42. Plenum Press, New York.

Plaas-Link, A. (1981). Die Wirkung von arteriellen P_{CO_2} oszillationen auf die atmung. PhD dissertation, Ruhr Universitat Bochum, Bochum, FRG.

Saunders, K. B. (1980). Oscillations of arterial CO_2 tension in a respiratory model: Some implications for the control of breathing in exercise. *Journal of Theoretical Biology*, **84**, 163–79.

Wasserman, K., Whipp, B. J. & Davis, J. A. (1981). Respiratory physiology of exercise. Metabolism, gas exchange and ventilatory control. In: *International Review of Physiology, Respiratory Physiology III*, vol. 23 (Widdicombe, J. G., ed.), pp. 149–211. University Park Press, Baltimore.

Weissman, M. L., Whipp, B. J., Huntsman, D. J. & Wasserman, K. (1980). Role of neural afferents from working limbs in exercise hyperpnea. *Journal of Applied Physiology*, **49**, 239–48.

Whipp, B. J. (1981). The control of the exercise hyperpnea. In: *Regulation of Breathing* (Hornbein, T. F., ed.) pp. 1069–139. Dekker, New York.

Yamamoto, W. S. (1960). Mathematical analysis of the time course of alveolar carbon dioxide. *Journal of Applied Physiology*, **15**, 315–19.

Yamamoto, W. S. & Edwards, M. W. (1960). Homeostasis of carbon dioxide during intravenous infusion of carbon dioxide. *Journal of Applied Physiology*, **15**, 807–18.

5

The control of exercise hyperpnoea

B. J. Whipp Division of Respiratory Physiology and Medicine, Harbor-UCLA Medical Center, Torrance

5.1 Introduction

The physiological mechanisms which control exercise hyperpnoea are manifestations of crucial evolutionary pressures for survival. It is not often recognised that were the alveolar ventilation ($\dot{V}_A$) of a standard (70 kg) subject to remain at resting level, it would not be possible to sustain the modest walking speed of 2.5 mph on a level surface without the alveolar PO_2 decreasing below that experienced by a free-breathing subject at the summit of Mount Everest; that is, below the limit for human survival.

It is perhaps surprising, therefore, that such a fundamental process is so poorly understood. This lack of understanding does not reflect a lack of proposed control mechanisms, but rather that the conclusions reached by different investigators from different experiments often suggest such contradictory and even, on occasion, mutually exclusive schemes of control; the challenge, therefore, is largely one of synthesis.

A meaningful analysis of ventilatory control during exercise (in this case, dynamic exercise performed under laboratory conditions at sea level) should utilise the rates of pulmonary gas exchange as a frame of reference; i.e. the rates of O_2 uptake ($\dot{V}_{O_2}$) and CO_2 output ($\dot{V}_{CO_2}$). Furthermore, it is convenient to consider three temporal and three intensity domains of exercise.

Temporal domains: **Phase 1 (φ1)** is the period between exercise onset and the beginning of change in the gas tensions (PCO_2, PO_2) in mixed venous blood which enters the pulmonary capillaries. The increased $\dot{V}_{O_2}$ and $\dot{V}_{CO_2}$ in this phase of the work are therefore a result of alterations of pulmonary blood flow ($\dot{Q}$) (and its distribution) and not a change of mixed venous blood composition. **Phase 2 (φ2)** is the subsequent dynamic phase in which the rates of pulmonary gas exchange are dictated by changing mixed venous blood composition, in addition to altered $\dot{Q}$. **Phase 3 (φ3)** is the steady state of the response.

Intensity domains: **Moderate** exercise may be considered to represent the range of work rates at which there is no sustained elevation of arterial blood lactate concentration $[La^-]_a$. **Heavy** exercise is that range in which there is a sustained elevation of $[La^-]_a$, with $[La^-]_a$ being maintained constant or even decreasing with time. **Severe** exercise represents those work rates for which $[La^-]_a$ continues to increase throughout the duration of the work, and results in fatigue consequent to the attainment of the subject's maximum $\dot{V}_{O_2}$.

5.2 Determinants of ventilation

A, and possibly the, major determinant for ventilation ($\dot{V}_E$) during exercise is the regulation of arterial blood gas (P_aO_2, P_aCO_2) and acid-base (pH_a) status. Consequently, the profiles of $\dot{V}_{O_2}$ and $\dot{V}_{CO_2}$ should be considered crucial frames of reference within which to judge the appropriateness of the ventilatory response. The general features of the $\dot{V}_E$ response to exercise are widely, though not unanimously, agreed upon: at moderate work rates, the normal subject increases $\dot{V}_E$ sufficiently to maintain P_aCO_2 and pH_a relatively constant. It is therefore useful to consider the quantitative interrelationships among those variables which establish this regulation.

In the ideal lung (one with no ventilation-perfusion inequalities, no diffusion limitation, no right-to-left shunt), alveolar and arterial PCO_2 are equal at a value which is determined by the ratio of $\dot{V}_{CO_2}$ to $\dot{V}_A$

$$P_ACO_2 = 863 \cdot \dot{V}_{CO_2}[\text{STPD}]/\dot{V}_A[\text{BTPS}] \qquad (5.1)$$

where P_ACO_2 is the CO_2 tension in alveolar gas; and 863 is the constant which derives from the necessary temperature, pressure and water vapour pressure corrections, owing to the conventions for reporting metabolic rate at standard temperature and pressure (dry) (STPD) and ventilation at body temperature and pressure (saturated) (BTPS); i.e., $[(273 + 37)/273] \cdot [760/(760 - 47)] \cdot (P_B - 47) = 863$. Thus

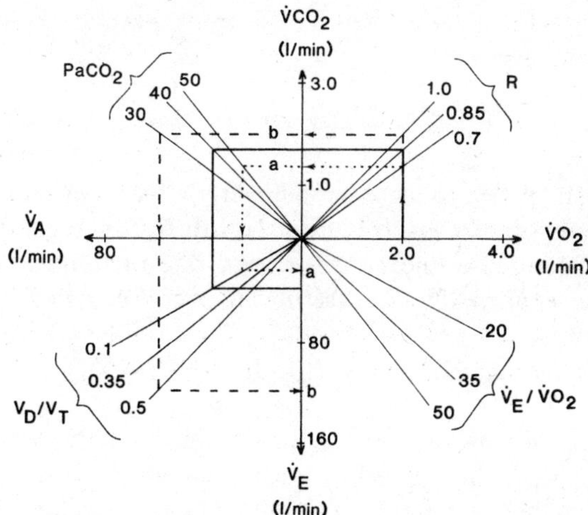

Fig. 5.1 Graphic display of influence of respiratory exchange ratio (R), arterial PCO_2 (P_aCO_2) and dead-space fraction of breath (V_D/V_T) on ventilatory requirement ($\dot{V}_E$) for exercise. For a particular O_2 uptake ($\dot{V}_{O_2}$), the $\dot{V}_E$ requirement can be significantly altered from normal response (solid line), with a particular combination of determining variables leading to a reduced (dotted line; arrow a) or markedly high (dashed line; arrow b) $\dot{V}_E$. (From Whipp & Pardy, 1986.)

$$P_aCO_2 = 863 \cdot \dot{V}_{CO_2}/\dot{V}_A \quad \text{or} \quad \dot{V}_A = 863 \cdot \dot{V}_{CO_2}/P_aCO_2 \quad (5.2)$$

Under conditions in which P_aCO_2 is maintained constant, the $\dot{V}_A$–$\dot{V}_{CO_2}$ relationship is therefore linear with a slope of 863/P_aCO_2 and passes through the origin (Figure 5.1, top left). Consequently – if P_aCO_2 is to be regulated – the lower the P_aCO_2, the greater must be the *increase* in $\dot{V}_A$ as work rate and $\dot{V}_{CO_2}$ rise during exercise. This would apply to a sea-level native sojourning at high altitude or a subject with a sustained metabolic acidosis, for example. Similarly, the higher the set-point P_aCO_2, the *less* will be the required increase in $\dot{V}_A$.

However, as the body ventilates not simply with alveolar ventilation but with total ventilation (i.e. each breath must also ventilate the dead space), we must also consider the $\dot{V}_E$–$\dot{V}_{CO_2}$ relationship during exercise. Two additional but related constructs therefore need to be considered: the dead space ventilation ($\dot{V}_D$) which reflects the size of the physiological dead space (V_D) multiplied by breathing frequency, and the ratio of dead space to tidal volume (V_D/V_T) which is the dead space fraction of the breath. From eqn (5.2)

$$\dot{V}_E = 863 \cdot \dot{V}_{CO_2}/P_aCO_2 + \dot{V}_D \qquad (5.3)$$

As the $\dot{V}_E$ response to incremental exercise has been shown to be a linear function of $\dot{V}_{CO_2}$ (Figure 5.2) with P_aCO_2 regulation, $\dot{V}_D$ must either increase linearly with work rate or remain constant. The former is normally the case during exercise. Alternatively,

$$\dot{V}_E = 863 \cdot \dot{V}_{CO_2}/P_aCO_2\,(1 - V_D/V_T) \qquad (5.4)$$

It is not intuitively obvious, at first sight, that the well-known linear $\dot{V}_E$–$\dot{V}_{CO_2}$ relationship during steady-state incremental exercise can be explained by this equation, as V_D/V_T is not a constant but rather decreases progressively with increasing work rate. However, the $\dot{V}_E$–$\dot{V}_{CO_2}$ relationship can still be linear under these conditions, with P_aCO_2 being regulated – but only if V_D/V_T falls as a hyperbolic function of increasing $\dot{V}_{CO_2}$ (Whipp & Ward, 1982)

$$V_D/V_T = 1 - [863 \cdot m/P_aCO_2] + [C/\dot{V}_{CO_2}] \qquad (5.5)$$

where m is the slope of the $\dot{V}_E$–$\dot{V}_{CO_2}$ relationship and c is its positive $\dot{V}_E$ intercept. This decrease in V_D/V_T during incremental exercise reflects both improved topographical distribution of lung perfusion and the relative compliance of the dead space region (approximately half of which is extrathoracic) compared with the alveolar gas exchange region of the lung. The practical consideration is, therefore, that in any individual having a large V_D/V_T (Figure 5.1), $\dot{V}_E$ will be higher than normal at any given level of

Fig. 5.2 (opposite) Representative relationships between ventilation ($\dot{V}_E$) and CO_2 output ($\dot{V}_{CO_2}$) during exercise in man, to illustrate the close correlation between these two variables under steady-state conditions (Wasserman *et al.*, 1967; Jones, 1973) and during the non-steady states of square-wave (Herxheimer & Kost, 1932; Wasserman & Whipp, 1983) and sinusoidal (Casaburi *et al.*, 1978; Miyamoto *et al.*, 1983) work-rate forcings. (From Whipp & Ward, 1985.)

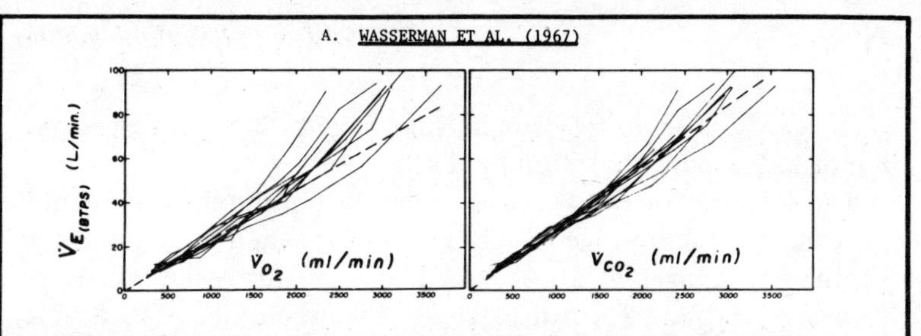
A. WASSERMAN ET AL. (1967)
$\dot{V}_{E(BTPS)}$ (L/min)
$\dot{V}_{O_2}$ (ml/min)
$\dot{V}_{CO_2}$ (ml/min)

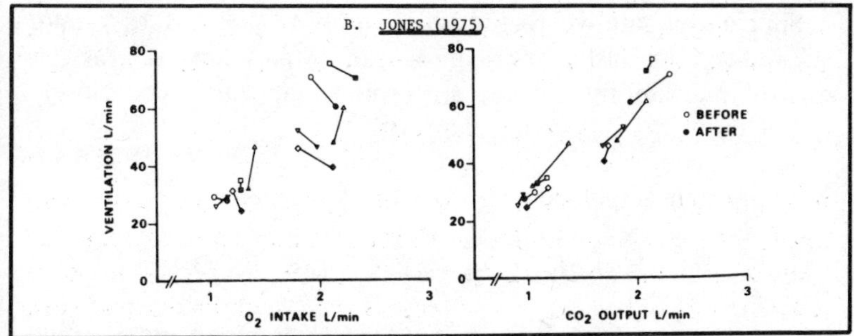
B. JONES (1975)
VENTILATION L/min
O_2 INTAKE L/min
CO_2 OUTPUT L/min
○ BEFORE
● AFTER

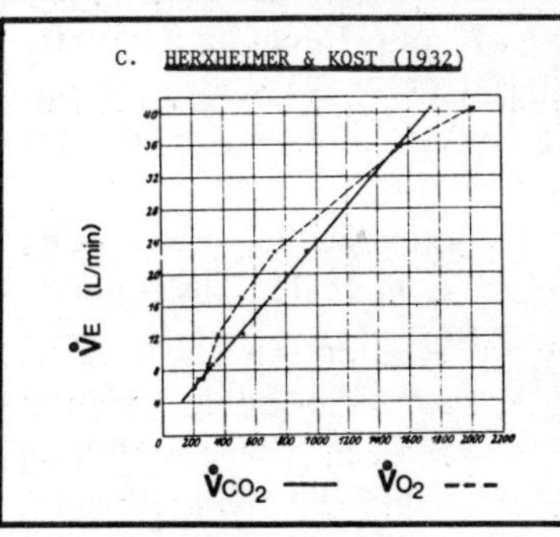
C. HERXHEIMER & KOST (1932)
$\dot{V}_E$ (L/min)
$\dot{V}_{CO_2}$ ——
$\dot{V}_{O_2}$ - - -

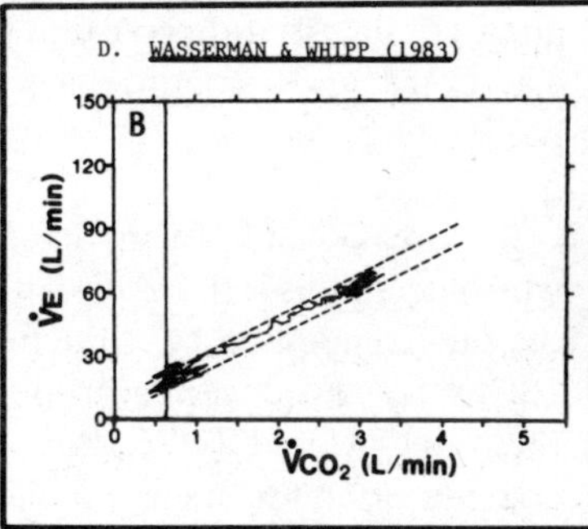
D. WASSERMAN & WHIPP (1983)
B
$\dot{V}_E$ (L/min)
$\dot{V}_{CO_2}$ (L/min)

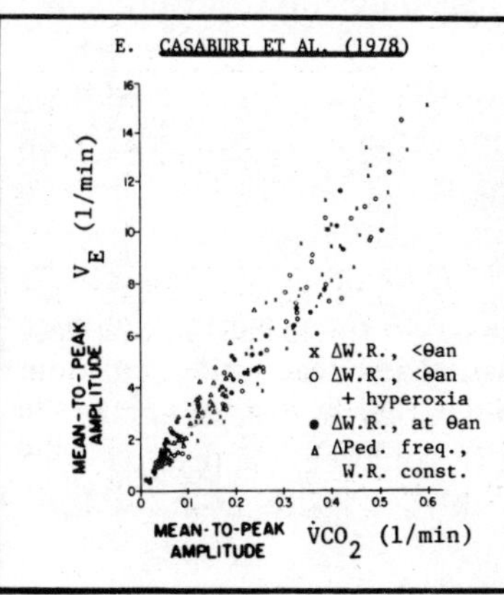
E. CASABURI ET AL. (1978)
MEAN-TO-PEAK AMPLITUDE V_E (1/min)
x ΔW.R., <θan
o ΔW.R., <θan + hyperoxia
● ΔW.R., at θan
▵ ΔPed. freq., W.R. const.
MEAN-TO-PEAK AMPLITUDE $\dot{V}CO_2$ (1/min)

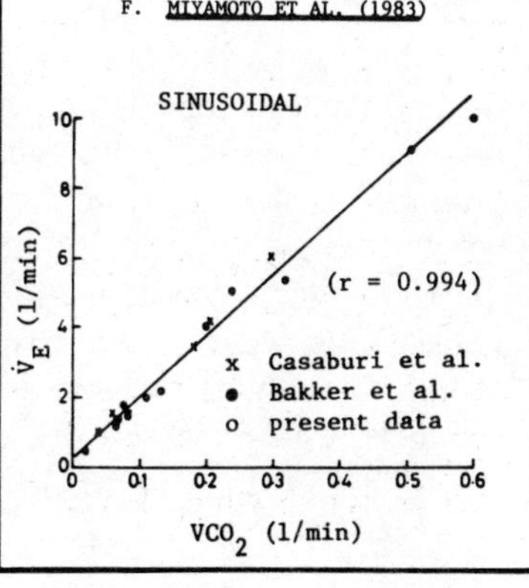
F. MIYAMOTO ET AL. (1983)
SINUSOIDAL
(r = 0.994)
$\dot{V}_E$ (1/min)
x Casaburi et al.
● Bakker et al.
o present data
VCO_2 (1/min)

$\dot{V}_{CO_2}$ if P_aCO_2 is to remain unchanged. This is especially important in patients with lung disease.

The linearity of the $\dot{V}_E$–$\dot{V}_{CO_2}$ relationship during incremental exercise and the positive $\dot{V}_E$ intercept ($3–5 l \cdot min^{-1}$) requires the ventilatory equivalent for CO_2 ($\dot{V}_E/\dot{V}_{CO_2}$ – this is the inverse of the mixed expired F_{CO_2}) to decrease hyperbolically as work rate and metabolic rate increase.

Similar quantitative relationships apply to $\dot{V}_E$ and $\dot{V}_{O_2}$. (We stress the relationship between $\dot{V}_E$ and $\dot{V}_{CO_2}$, however, as the control mechanisms for the hyperpnoea appear to be closely correlated with $\dot{V}_{CO_2}$ rather than with $\dot{V}_{O_2}$).

The regulation of P_{a,CO_2} during moderate exercise, of course, has important implications for pH_a:

$$pH_a = pK' + \log ([HCO_3^-]_a/\alpha \cdot P_aCO_2) \qquad (5.6)$$

where α is the solubility coefficient for CO_2 in blood and K' is the apparent dissociation constant (with a pK' of 6.1 in human blood). Therefore, under conditions in which $[HCO_3^-]_a$ is not altered (i.e. moderate exercise), pH_a will remain constant only if P_aCO_2 does not change.

For heavy and severe exercise, a metabolic acidosis ensues which decreases $[HCO_3^-]_a$. The degree to which pH_a falls depends on the compensatory reduction in P_aCO_2. For example, were P_aCO_2 to be reduced in proportion to the decrease in $[HCO_3^-]_a$, then pH_a would be returned to normal (i.e. full respiratory compensation for the metabolic acidosis). Such full compensation, however, is not often seen and then only for relatively small degrees of metabolic acidosis (Wasserman *et al.*, 1967).

In the steady state of moderate exercise, the CO_2 evolved from the body reflects the mitochondrial formation of CO_2. But at work rates which result in an increased $[La^-]_a$, the CO_2 which is produced is derived from two additional sources. Firstly, some 90–95% of the buffering of the lactic acid produced is effected by the CO_2–HCO_3^- system; these buffering mechanisms therefore release CO_2 which is additional to that produced metabolically. Were $\dot{V}_E$ only to change in production to the metabolically produced CO_2 at these work rates, it would be inappropriate for the total CO_2 load and P_aCO_2 would rise resulting in an acute metabolic acidosis combined with a respiratory acidosis. However, were $\dot{V}_E$ to increase in proportion to the total CO_2 delivered to the lungs, then P_aCO_2 would be regulated at its control level; but there would be no respiratory compensation for the metabolic acidosis. In order to constrain the fall of pH_a at these work rates, P_aCO_2 needs to be *lowered* by the process of hyperventilation, which provides the third source of CO_2 evolved in high-intensity exercise.

Ventilatory control and the requirements for pH_a regulation therefore depend upon an interaction of three determining variables, viz., $\dot{V}_{CO_2}$, P_aCO_2 and V_D/V_T. This interaction is illustrated by the examples presented in Figure 5.1 which considers two subjects (*a, b*) who are exercising at the same steady state $\dot{V}_{O_2}$ ($2\ l \cdot min^{-1}$).

First, we assume that the subjects oxidise different substrates: a fatty acid (i.e., palmitic) with a respiratory quotient or 'metabolic exchange ratio' (*RQ*) and a respiratory exchange ratio or 'pulmonary exchange ratio' (*R*, or $\dot{V}_{CO_2}/\dot{V}_{O_2}$) of about 0.7 for subject *a*,; and carbohydrate (*RQ* & $R = 1.0$) for subject *b*. The corresponding values of $\dot{V}_{CO_2}$ are thus 1.4 and 2.0 $l \cdot min^{-1}$, respectively (upper right quadrant).

Next, we assume subject *a* to be moderately hypoventilating ($P_aCO_2 = 50$ mmHg) but with normal lung function and hence a normal V_D/V_T of 0.1 at this work rate. Combining the effects of a low $\dot{V}_{CO_2}$ (because of the low *R*) with a slightly elevated P_aCO_2 requires $\dot{V}_A$ to be $\sim 24\ l \cdot min^{-1}$ (upper left quadrant) which, with the normal V_D/V_T, yields a total $\dot{V}_E$ requirement of $\sim 27 l^{-1}$ (lower left quadrant).

In contrast, subject *b* – representative of a patient with pulmonary vascular occlusive disease or severe chronic obstructive pulmonary disease, for example – has a P_aCO_2 of 30 mmHg and an elevated V_D/V_T of 0.5; both of which 'conspire' with the high $\dot{V}_{CO_2}$ (because of the high *R*) to raise the total $\dot{V}_E$ requirement to $\sim 115\ l \cdot min^{-1}$.

These greater than four-fold differences in ventilatory requirement for the same exercise $\dot{V}_{O_2}$ emphasise the importance of the determinants of exercise $\dot{V}_E$ and the extent to which they require responses that may encroach on the mechanical and metabolic limits of the system. This is particularly important in patients with chronic obstructive pulmonary disease, for example, in whom the maximum attainable level of $\dot{V}_E$ is markedly reduced or in highly fit athletes who are capable of developing extremely high levels of metabolic rate.

5.3 **Ventilatory response characteristics**

It is important that the characteristic features of the $\dot{V}_E$ response to exercise both be clearly recognised and used as the yardstick by which the appropriateness of a proposed control mechanism is assessed.

5.3.1 *Steady-state responses: moderate exercise*

For steady-state increments of work rate, $\dot{V}_E$ increases more linearly with respect to $\dot{V}_{CO_2}$ than to $\dot{V}_{O_2}$ (Wasserman *et al.*, 1967). In addition, when subjects undergo endurance training, such that the post-training $\dot{V}_{CO_2}$ at the given work load is less than that prior to training, $\dot{V}_E$ is decreased in rather precise proportion to the CO_2 that was *not* produced at these workloads following training (Figure 5.2); in contrast, there appears to be no direct relationship between the decrement in $\dot{V}_E$ and the change in $\dot{V}_{O_2}$ (Jones, 1975). Furthermore, the regulated level of resting P_aCO_2 can be altered by means of sustained diet-induced metabolic acidosis and alkalosis (Jones & Haddon, 1973; Oren *et al.*, 1981): $\dot{V}_E$ was affected during moderate exercise precisely as predicted for regulation of P_aCO_2 with an altered 'set-point' – see eqn (5.3).

P_aCO_2 is therefore regulated at or close to its control level during the steady state, as a result of the close matching between $\dot{V}_E$ and $\dot{V}_{CO_2}$. (However, care must be taken not to misinterpret an increase in P_aCO_2 between rest and exercise that can often result from subsequent correction of the hyperventilation which many subjects manifest when initially connected to the breathing apparatus.) This suggests that in general – by whatever mechanism – the exercise hyperpnoea is likely to be linked to a mechanism proportional to pulmonary CO_2 exchange.

Other investigators, however, do not find evidence such as that presented in Figure 5.2 to be sufficiently convincing for a necessary CO_2-linkage in the exercise hyperpnoea. Fordyce & Bennett (1984), using mathematical modelling, have questioned whether the demonstrated regulation of P_aCO_2 during exercise necessarily implies the existence of a precise coupling between $\dot{V}_E$ and metabolic rate; while Dempsey *et al.* (1984) have actually questioned whether P_aCO_2 is a regulated variable. But there is a large body of literature which demonstrates that in the steady state (a crucial requirement) of moderate exercise in a quiet, non-threatening environment, P_aCO_2 is regulated at or close to the resting control value (see Whipp, 1981 for detailed discussion), although – as Dempsey *et al.* (1984) point out – this is usually based upon the mean responses of a group of subjects. Intriguingly, Poon (1983) has recently suggested a control scheme by which the regulated level of P_aCO_2 during exercise might result from an optimisation strategy incorporating both CO_2-responsiveness and the work of breathing. The functional significance of this interesting scheme, however, remains to be established experimentally.

Care should be taken, however, not to misinterpret increases in end-tidal PCO_2 ($P_{ET}CO_2$) as a necessary manifestation of increases in P_aCO_2. For example, as the pulmonary CO_2 flux (i.e. the product of pulmonary blood flow and mixed venous CO_2 content) increases progressively with work rate, the slope of the alveolar phase of expired PCO_2 consequently also rises. This results in $P_{ET}CO_2$ increasing (Figures 5.3 and 5.4) in proportion to $\dot{V}_{CO_2}$ to values above the effectively unaltered mean P_aCO_2.

5.3.2 *Steady-state responses: heavy and severe exercise*

Above the threshold $\dot{V}_{O_2}$ at which a sustained lactic acidosis ensues (also known as the **anaerobic threshold**, θ_{an}: Wasserman & McIlroy, 1964), the $\dot{V}_E$ response becomes highly non-linear and with steady states commonly unattainable. The acidaemia provides additional $\dot{V}_E$ drive which effects a reduction in P_aCO_2 as respiratory compensation for the acidosis.

In response to incremental exercise of a quasi-steady-state nature (i.e. increment durations > 4 min), $\dot{V}_E$ increases at a progressively faster rate relative to work rate and $\dot{V}_{O_2}$ above θ_{an} than for moderate-intensity exercise (Figure 5.2; also evident in Figures 5.4 and 5.5). A correspondingly more marked rate of increase is also evident in $\dot{V}_{CO_2}$, reflecting that above θ_{an} the delivery of metabolically-produced CO_2 to the lungs is supple-

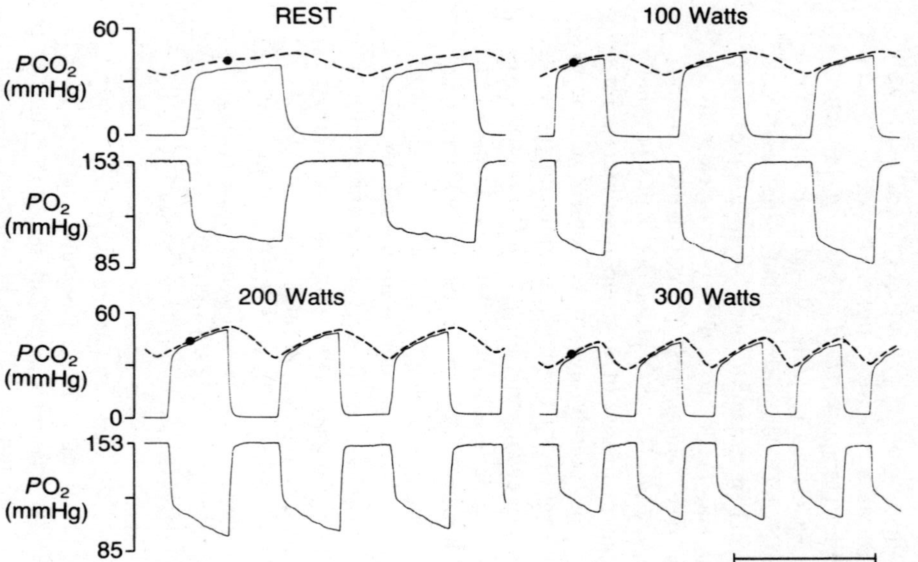

Fig. 5.3 Breath-by-breath profiles of respired PCO_2 and PO_2 at rest and during exercise (100, 200 and 300 W) in man to illustrate the progressive steepening of the slope of the expiratory alveolar phase with increasing work rate. An estimated profile of arterial PCO_2 has been superimposed (dashed lines) to characterise its respiratory-related oscillation. Note that while mean P_aCO_2 (●) is stable, there is (with the exception of the resting condition) a progressive increase in end-tidal PCO_2 above this value as work rate increases. (From Whipp, 1977, *Exercise and Sport Sciences Reviews*, Vol. 5, Fig. 5, p. 303. Copyright 1977, American College of Sports Medicine. Reproduced by permission.)

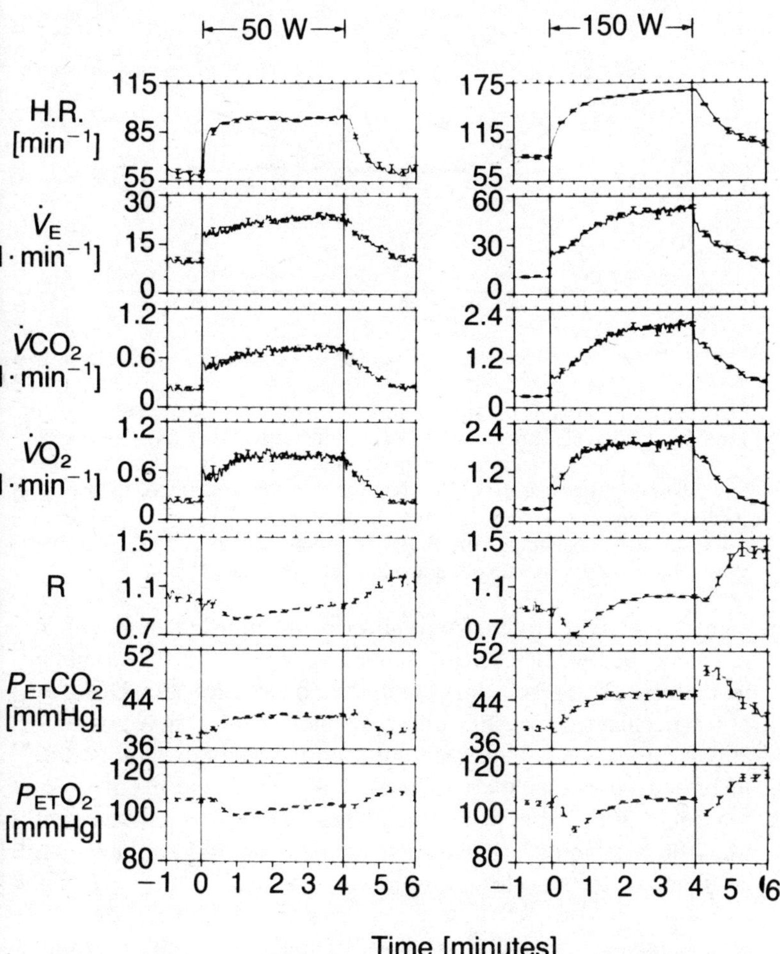

Fig. 5.4 Mean ($n = 8$) breath-by-breath ventilatory and gas-exchange responses to a step-increase of work rate (50 W, left panels; 150 W, right panels) from rest in a single subject. Note the stability of $P_{ET}CO_2$, $P_{ET}O_2$ and R across the rest-exercise transition, the transient undershoot of R and $P_{ET}O_2$ starting at *ca* 20 s, and the subsequent slower uprise of $\dot{V}_E$, $\dot{V}_{CO_2}$ and $\dot{V}_{O_2}$ to their new steady states. (From Wasserman *et al.*, 1986.)

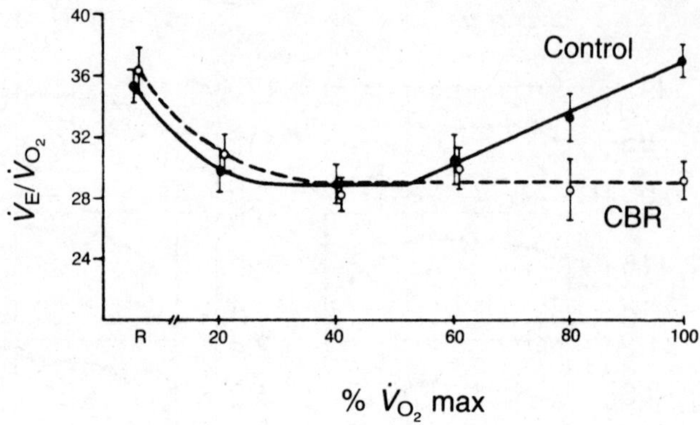

Fig. 5.5 Comparison of the ventilatory response (expressed as the ventilatory equivalent for O_2, $\dot{V}_E/\dot{V}_{O_2}$) to incremental exercise between a control group of subjects and a group that previously had both carotid bodies surgically resected (CBR). Note that in the control group, $\dot{V}_E/\dot{V}_{O_2}$ started to increase at ca. 50%–60% of maximal $\dot{V}_{O_2}$ ($\dot{V}_{O_2}$ max), while this response was absent in the CBR subjects (----). (From Whipp & Wasserman, 1980, courtesy 'Federation Proceedings'.)

mented by CO_2 deriving from buffering reactions (see above). As discussed below, the carotid bodies appear to be the dominant mediators of this respiratory compensation (Figure 5.5). However, other mechanisms which could supplement the $\dot{V}_E$ drive above θ_{an} may include catecholamines, a sufficiently high body temperature, increased blood osmolarity, arterial K^+ ions, and even anxiety regarding the high work load. For example, patients with McArdle's syndrome – who are unable to produce lactic acid consequent to muscle phosphorylase B deficiency – actually develop a marked respiratory alkalosis at a relatively low work rate (equivalent to 50% or more of their (reduced) maximum capacity: Hagberg *et al.*, 1982).

However, when the work rate is incremented rapidly (in 1-min stages, or less), $\dot{V}_E$ actually retains its sub-θ_{an} proportionality to $\dot{V}_{CO_2}$ over a substantial portion of the supra-θ_{an} range (see Cunningham, 1974; Whipp, 1981). Thus, there appears to be no corresponding increase in the ventilatory equivalent for CO_2 ($\dot{V}_E/\dot{V}_{CO_2}$) or decrease in $P_{ET}CO_2$ until a point approximately half-way between θ_{an} and maximum is attained. This domain of work rate has been termed the range of 'isocapnic buffering'

(Wasserman *et al.*, 1977). The functional basis for this unusual pattern of response (i.e. hyperventilation relative to O_2, but not to CO_2) is presently uncertain. The carotid bodies may not be immediately responsive to a falling pH_a, consequent perhaps to the existence of some amplitude- or time-related threshold for excitation by H^+ ions.

5.3.3 *Dynamic responses*

As for any control system, the most important features of its behaviour can only be deduced from its transient response characteristics. We shall therefore consider the non-steady-state phases of the exercise hyperpnoea.

5.3.3.1 *Phase 1 (φ1).* Krogh & Lindhard (1913) were the first to document systematically that a 'rapid' hyperpnoea occurred at exercise onset (see e.g., Figure 5.4). This response occurs in virtual synchrony with the onset of the work and can begin in either the inspiratory or expiratory phase of the respiratory cycle (if cued by a preparatory warning, the ventilatory changes may even precede the exercise). The magnitude of this initial increment of $\dot{V}_E$ is relatively constant, irrespective of the work rate, and lasts for some 20 s. The dynamics of the early $\dot{V}_E$ response depend, however, upon whether the constant-load work is imposed from a background or rest or of mild exercise: in the latter situation, a more slowly developing hyperpnoea results (Figures 5.6 and 5.7).

Recently, dynamic work-rate forcing techniques and computer analysis have detailed the response characteristics of φ1. Forcings include the square wave and its integral and differential (i.e. the ramp and impulse functions, respectively), pseudo-random binary sequences, and sinusoidal functions. These studies provide support that the $\dot{V}_E$ response is two-phased, even against a background of prior mild exercise.

An important feature of the φ1 hyperpnoea is that if the rest-to-work transition is instituted with the subject in the supine rather than the upright posture, there is no rapid φ1 component; rather, the response resembles that for the work-to-work transition of upright exercise (Karlsson *et al.*, 1975; Weiler-Ravell *et al.*, 1983).

Several groups have demonstrated that the φ1 hyperpnoea is

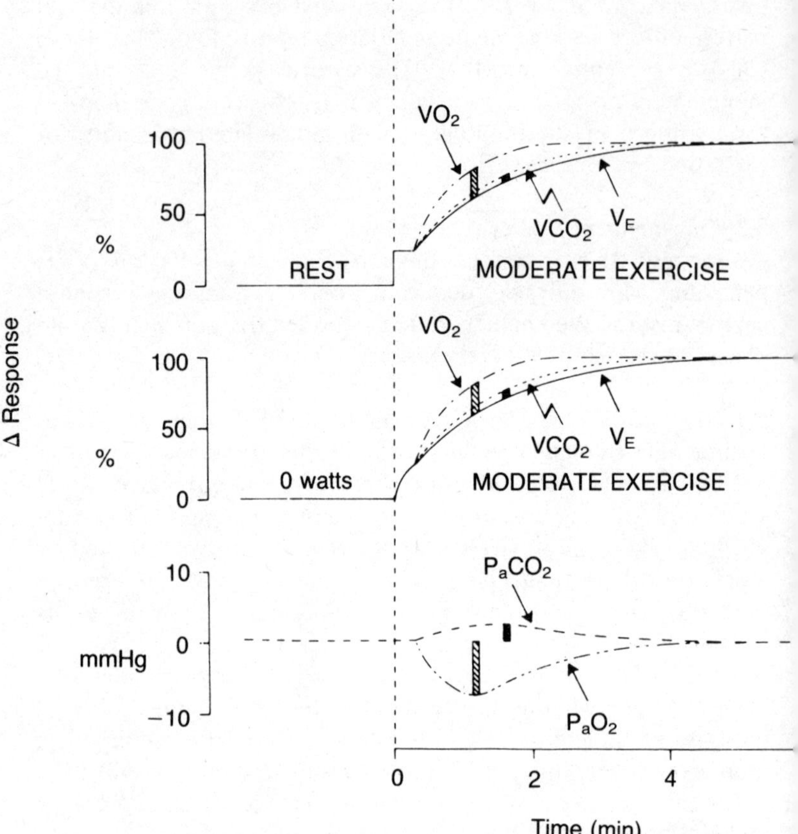

Fig. 5.6 Schematic representation of time course of ventilation ($\dot{V}_E$), CO_2 output ($\dot{V}_{CO_2}$) and O_2 uptake ($\dot{V}_{O_2}$) in response to a moderate step increase of work rate from rest (top) or from unloaded pedalling (middle), and of arterial PCO_2 and PO_2 (bottom). Vertical bars indicate occurrence of maximal temporal dissociation of $\dot{V}_E$ from gas exchange response, coincident with maximal arterial blood gas derangement: CO_2 (solid bars), O_2 (hatched bars). (From Whipp & Ward 1980, 'Ventilatory control dynamics during muscular exercise in man', *International Journal of Sports Medicine* 1: 146–59.)

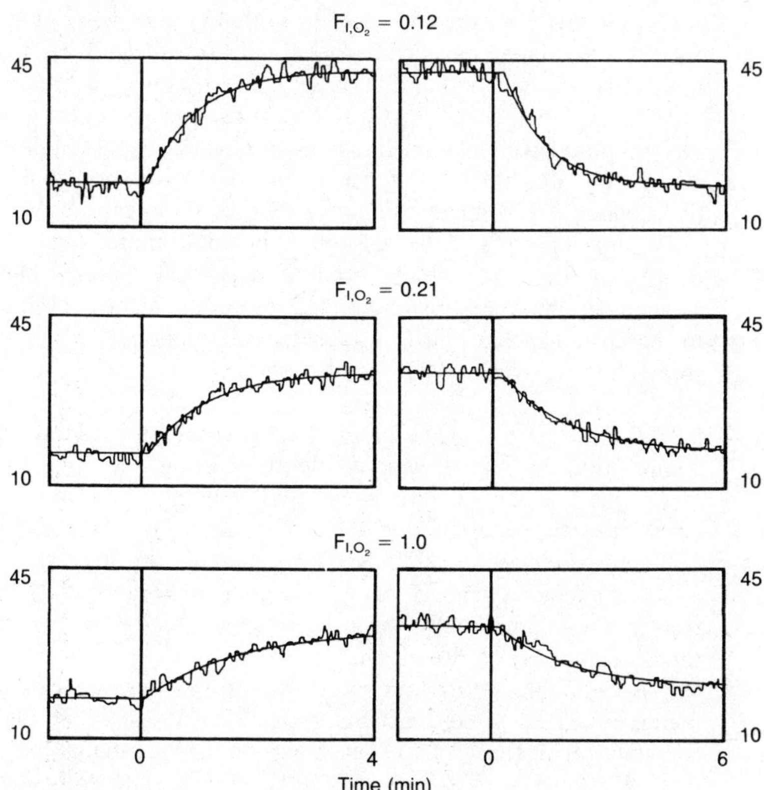

Fig. 5.7 Mean (n = 4) breath-by-breath ventilatory ($\dot{V}_E$) response to a moderate step-increase of work rate from unloaded pedalling in a single subject, against backgrounds of differing inhaled O_2 fraction (F_IO_2). Note the speeding of the response dynamics as F_IO_2 is lowered from 1.0 to 0.12. (From Griffiths *et al.*, 1986.)

typically not associated with the increase in the respiratory exchange ratio R and $P_{ET}O_2$ and the decrease in $P_{ET}CO_2$ characteristic of hyperventilation (see, e.g., Figure 5.4), although others have reported hyperventilation at exercise onset (see Whipp, 1981 for further discussion).

As R and the end-tidal gas tensions – and presumably, therefore, P_aCO_2 and P_aO_2 – often remain relatively stable across the transition and the initial hyperpnoea is accompanied by correspondingly abrupt increases in both $\dot{V}_{O_2}$ and $\dot{V}_{CO_2}$ (Figure 5.4), this precludes specific neurogenic control *solely* of $\dot{V}_E$ in φ1; this would elicit hyperventilation with a consequent decrease of $P_{ET}CO_2$ and increase of $P_{ET}O_2$ and R. Consequently, as the mixed venous blood composition has not yet changed, the stability of R and the end-tidal gas tensions in φ1 is evidence that the hyperpnoea is accompanied by a proportional increase in $\dot{Q}$.

This inference raised the possibility that either there is an abrupt neurogenic drive to both $\dot{V}_E$ and $\dot{Q}$ at exercise onset – inconsequent simultaneity – or that the $\dot{V}_E$ response may be consequent to the abrupt increase in Q – causal cardiopulmonary coupling – (see Whipp & Ward, 1982, for discussion).

5.3.3.2 *Phase 2 (φ2)*. The onset of φ2 is signalled by altered gas composition in mixed venous blood entering the pulmonary capillaries – a phenomenon suggestive of humoral control. This accelerates the rates of transfer of O_2 and CO_2 across the gas exchange interface and leads to an increase in $P_{ET}CO_2$ and a simultaneous decrease of $P_{ET}O_2$ and R (Figure 5.4). $\dot{V}_E$ rises mono-exponentially towards the new steady state with a time constant (τ) of 70 s or so.

It is clear that – for work rates which do not evoke sustained increases of $[La^-]_a$ – the dynamic reponses of $\dot{V}_E$ in φ2 are highly correlated with those of CO_2 exchange (not O_2 exchange) at the lung (Figure 5.2): $\dot{V}_{O_2}$ increases to its steady state with a τ of 30–40 s, whereas $\dot{V}_{CO_2}$ responds much more slowly (τ ca. 60–70 s). The kinetic dissociation of $\dot{V}_{O_2}$ and $\dot{V}_{CO_2}$ in φ2 predominantly reflects the influence of the intervening body gas stores: the body's CO_2 capacitance is substantially greater than for O_2. Consequently, some of the metabolically produced CO_2 is stored during the transient and is therefore not exchanged at the lungs; $\dot{V}_E$ therefore appears to change during φ2 with a time course which resembles that of the pulmonary exchange rate of CO_2 rather than its rate of metabolic production.

As a consequence of τ $\dot{V}_E$ being appreciably longer than τ $\dot{V}_{O_2}$, P_aO_2 falls transiently during φ2 (Young & Woolcock, 1978; Oldenburg *et al.*, 1979) (Figure 5.6). In contrast, the relatively small kinetic dissociation between $\dot{V}_E$ and $\dot{V}_{CO_2}$ in φ2 (e.g. Casaburi *et al.*, 1977) leads to the transient increase expected for

P_aCO_2 to be rather small (Figure 5.6); at present, it has only been discerned in response to multiple repetitions of sinusoidal exercise (Whipp, 1981).

5.4 **Proposed control mechanisms**

Current proposals which purport to account for exercise hyperpnoea involve, to varying degrees of exclusivity, neurogenic and humoral mechanisms.

5.4.1 *Neural control*

As the immediacy of the $\dot{V}_E$ response to exercise appears incompatible with a humorally mediated drive from metabolites released from the working limbs stimulating known sites of chemoreception (i.e. the carotid bodies and the ventral medullary surface), neurogenic mechanisms originating in the exercising limbs and/or suprabulbar regions have been proposed to account for the φ1 hyperpnoea.

An involvement of muscle reflexogenic drive is supported by evidence from several sources. If the somatic afferent projections from the hind limbs of anaesthetised cats or dogs (induced to exercise by electrical stimulation of the appropriate motor nerves or of the muscles themselves) are interrupted by complete spinal section or lateral-column section (Kao, 1963) or by blockade of afferent fibers from the exercising limbs (McCloskey & Mitchell, 1972; Tibes, 1977), the neurogenic component of exercise hyperpnoea has been shown to be abolished.

But evidence suggestive of parallel activation of both cardiovascular and $\dot{V}_E$ responses is also available. When the afferent traffic in the group III and group IV somatic projections from the exercising hind limbs of the cat were interrupted, not only was the hyperpnoeic response to the work largely abolished but so were the associated cardiovascular responses (McCloskey & Mitchell, 1972).

Although an involvement of muscle spindles in the control of the φ1 hyperpnoea has been suggested – largely as a result of pharmacological studies – blockade of the large myelinated fibers however has little or no effect. This notion is supported by the demonstration that high frequency, low amplitude vibration of the hind limb muscles (a potent muscle spindle stimulus) has little effect on $\dot{V}_E$ in the cat (Hodgson & Matthews, 1968). Furthermore, in man selective blockade of the gamma efferent projections to the muscle spindles of the legs by infiltration of the lower lumbar peridural space with lidocaine had no effect on the development of the exercise hyperpnoea.

Tibes (1977) has also argued for peripheral neural control of the φ2 hyperpnoea, because of the close temporal correlation observed in the non-steady-state between $\dot{V}_E$ and $[K^+]$ in the venous effluent from the exercising muscles (a stimulant of non-myelinated muscle afferents – and the carotid bodies, it has subsequently been shown: Band *et al.*, 1985). This proposal, although in agreement with the results of Kao (1963), is not consistent with the more recent observations of Weissman *et al.* (1979) and Cross *et al.* (1982), who demonstrated that interruption of somatic afferent traffic from the exercising limbs had no discernible effect on the kinetics of the φ2 hyperpnoea, especially when related to the corresponding $\dot{V}_{CO_2}$ response. Also, the time course of the $\dot{V}_E$ response to electrically induced exercise in patients with complete thoracic or lumbar spinal cord transection did not differ from that of spinally-intact control subjects (Adams *et al.*, 1984; Brice *et al.*, 1986; and Chapter 4 of this book.). An earlier study by Asmussen *et al.* (1943) had also shown the steady-state $\dot{V}_E$ response to exercise was essentially normal in a subject with tabes dorsalis who had complete loss of proprioceptive reflexes from the legs and lower trunk.

Furthermore, as the magnitude of the φ1 hyperpnoea (from rest) is relatively constant despite progressively greater imposed work loads (Dejours, 1964; Jensen, 1972) (and a much slower rate of change results from a background of unloaded pedalling or at the onset of supine exercise), the change in $\dot{V}_E$ is not simply proportional to the recruitment of motor units or to the imposed work load.

Krogh & Lindhard (1913) suggested that descending activity from areas controlling limb motion 'irradiated' to bulbar respiratory and cardiovascular centres to evoke increases in $\dot{V}_E$ and $\dot{Q}$ synchronously with exercise onset. This contention has support in the hyperventilation which has been observed during steady-state exercise under conditions in which the degree of conscious effort required to accomplish a specific motor task was caused to be greater than normal; e.g. following partial muscle curarisation (Asmussen *et al.*, 1965), by hypnotic suggestion (Daly & Overly, 1966; Morgan *et al.*, 1973) and by simultaneous activation of antagonistic musculature (Goodwin *et al.*, 1972). In contrast, a strong argument against an involvement of cortical structures in the hyperpnoea derives from the observation by Dejours *et al.* (1959) that light general anaesthesia had little effect on the magnitude of the initial $\dot{V}_E$ response to passive leg exercise, and also that the time course of the hyperpnoea in response to electrically induced muscle contractions in normal and spinally transected subjects was not appreciably different from volitionally-induced exercise (see above).

Evidence for a coupling between descending pathways for limb locomotor and ventilatory (i.e. thoracic locomotor) activity has been demonstrated by Eldridge *et al.* (1985) (this is an indispensible article for consideration of the neural control of the exercise hyperpnoea); among other experimental procedures, these authors stimulated the 'hypothalamic motor area' electrically in the cat. However, there was a striking fall in $P_{ET}CO_2$ in these experiments which is in marked contrast to the isocapnia or small hypocapnia typically observed in φ1 of volitional exercise in man; but this may be characteristic of the cat.

It has been further pointed out that the slowness of φ2 hyperpnoea should not be used as a necessary basis for precluding neural involvement in its mediation – in the same sense that Wasserman *et al.* (1974) cautioned that the rapidity of the φ1 hyperpnoea does not preclude a humorally induced control (see below). Eldridge (1977) thus demonstrated that neural 'reverberation' within the brainstem respiratory centres may induce a slowly-developing ventilatory response following an abrupt change in respiratory stimulus. That is, the sudden reduction of afferent drive to the respiratory centres (via stimulation of the carotid bodies, the central chemoreceptor complex, or the hind-limb musculature of the cat) yielded a slowly-declining component of $\dot{V}_E$ to the new steady state which lasted several minutes. However, complicating a simple interpretation of these results, the mechanism is not as evident at an on-transient of stimulation, whereas the dynamics of the φ2 hyperpnoea in man are symmetrical for on- and off-responses (Casaburi *et al.*, 1977; Griffiths *et al.*, 1986).

As described above, conditions associated with a rapid increase of $\dot{Q}$ at exercise onset (brought about by an abrupt rise of stroke volume) result in rapid hyperpnoea of relatively constant magnitude which is proportional to the magnitude of the $\dot{Q}$ response. This response is virtually unaltered by breathing air, hypoxic, hyperoxic or hypercapnic gas mixtures. However, when there is a slower, more gradual increase in $\dot{Q}$ at exercise onset because the stroke volume is already at, or near the exercising value (i.e. for work-to-work transitions, or for supine rest-to-work transitions), there is no rapid $\dot{V}_E$ response to the work.

The different dynamic response patterns of $\dot{V}_E$ have suggested to some investigators (Wasserman *et al.*, 1974) that there may be a direct link from the cardiovascular change which is responsible for the hyperpnoea (i.e. a 'cardiodynamic hyperpnoea'), rather than there being a 'parallel activiation' of both cardiovascular and ventilatory control systems which results in proportional increases in both $\dot{Q}$ and $\dot{V}_E$.

In an attempt to elucidate possible mechanical mechanisms of the proposed cardiodynamic hyperpnoea, Jones *et al.* (1982) and Huszczuk *et al.* (1983) manipulated the pressure in the right side of the heart by partial occlusion of the pulmonary artery outflow tract with a balloon. These investigators demonstrated an excellent correlation between the magnitude and profile of the right ventricular moving-average pressure and that of the $\dot{V}_E$ response which was not abolished by vagotomy. As a result, they proposed that afferents from the right ventricle may play a role in coupling $\dot{V}_E$ to cardiovascular changes under conditions such as exercise. Direct neurophysiological studies of hyperpnoea mediated by cardiac sympathetic afferents (Kostreva *et al.*, 1975; Uchida, 1976) provide a plausible pathway for such a mechanism.

Recently, Lloyd (1984) has used an isolated subsystem in dog that included both the right heart and the major pulmonary arteries, within which the pressure could be experimentally altered. Modest breathing frequency increases were observed when the system pressure was increased (range: 30–70 mmHg or 4.0–9.3 kPa) that were abolished by bilateral vagotomy. This led Lloyd to conclude that the sensitivity of this mechanism was likely to be too small to account for the results of Jones *et al.* (1982). However, when blood flow to the heart and lungs is reduced, by means of partial venous-to-arterial bypass and extracorporeal gas exchange, reductions of $\dot{V}_E$ have been consistently reported (Figure 5.8) supporting the suggestions of intrathoracic sensing mechanisms (Levine, 1978; Green & Sheldon, 1983; Huszczuk *et al.*, 1986*a*; Trenchard, 1986).

Jones *et al.* (1981) induced rapid increases of heart rate in patients (who had permanent demand-type pacemakers for the management of atrioventricular block). When the rate was increased abruptly from 50 to 80 min^{-1}, there was no significant response in $\dot{V}_E$ for about 20 s, despite $\dot{V}_{O_2}$, $\dot{V}_{CO_2}$ and $P_{ET}CO_2$ having increased and $P_{ET}O_2$ and R having decreased. Thus, $\dot{Q}$ appeared to be increased without a consequent increase in $\dot{V}_E$. The subsequent increase in $\dot{V}_E$, after the delay, presumably resulted fom humoral stimulation of the chemoreceptors by the altered blood gas tensions.

In summary, mechanisms originating in the heart and pulmonary vasculature have been documented as leading to ventilatory stimulation but the few direct studies on such a mechanism have produced not entirely consistent results. Recently, however, convincing evidence that cardiac-mediated mechanisms are not necessary for a normal hyperpnoeic response to exercise and consequent homeostasis of arterial blood gas and acid-base status has been furnished by experiments in humans who had undergone cardiac transplantation (Theodore *et al.*, 1986) and in the awake calf with an artifical (Jarvik-type) heart (Huszczuk *et al.*, 1986*b*).

5.4.2 *Humoral Control*

Eldridge and his associates (1985) concluded that 'even though central command signals provide much of the drive for adjustments of respiration and circulation, a number of feedback mechanisms may be involved in their fine control. They are probably responsible for the close tracking of ventilation and metabolic events during exercise'. The suggestion of humoral feedback control of exercise hyperpnoea is usually based upon observations that:

(a) the slower φ2 response only begins after a delay which is commensurate with the transit delay from the exercising limbs

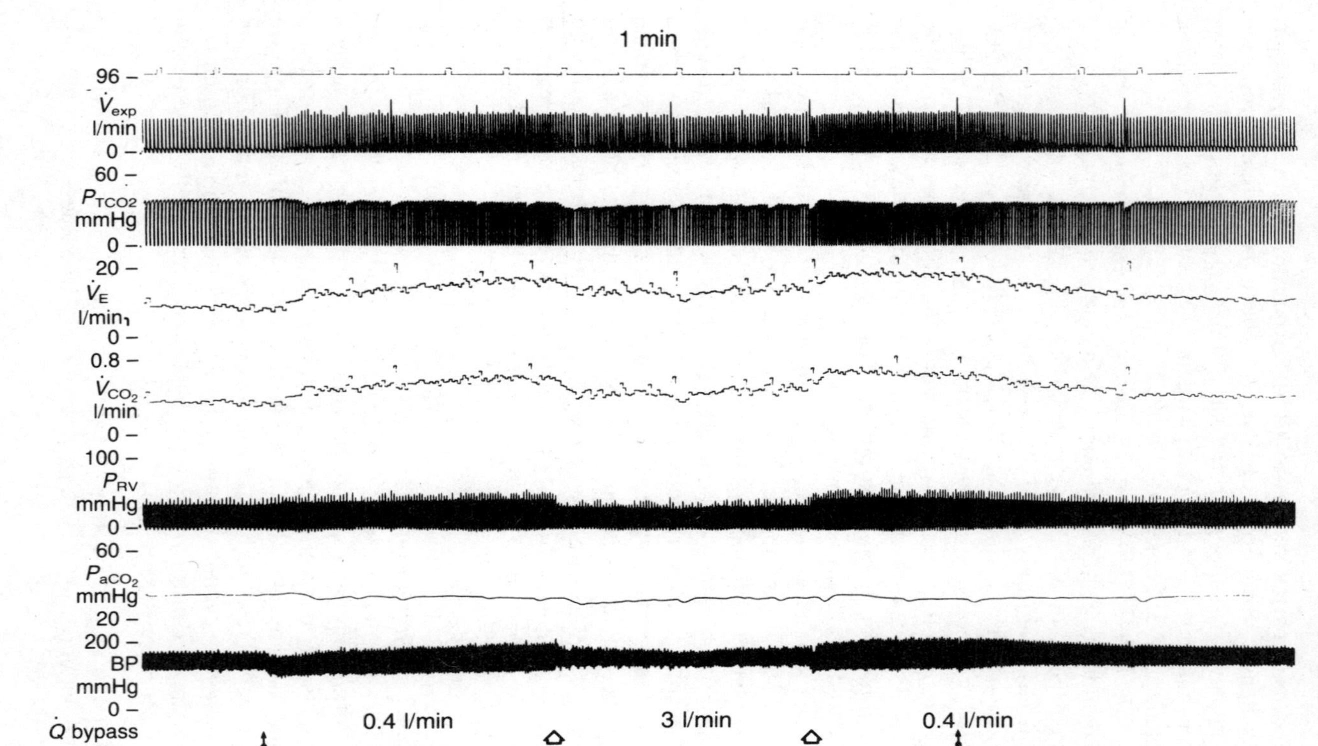
1 min
96 –
$\dot{V}_{exp}$
l/min
0 –
60 –
P_{TCO2}
mmHg
0 –
20 –
$\dot{V}_E$
l/min
0 –
0.8 –
$\dot{V}_{CO_2}$
l/min
0 –
100 –
P_{RV}
mmHg
0 –
60 –
P_{aCO_2}
mmHg
20 –
200 –
BP
mmHg
0 –
$\dot{Q}$ bypass
0.4 l/min
3 l/min
0.4 l/min

to the lungs – or some structure located in close, downstream proximity;

(b) the subsequent dynamic $\dot{V}_E$ response pattern is so closely related to the time course of the pulmonary CO_2 exchange;

(c) in the steady state, P_aCO_2 and pH_a appear to be regulated at, or close to, the control (i.e. 'set-point') values.

And, of course, under conditions in which mean P_aCO_2 increases during exercise, $\dot{V}_E$ is not usually increased in response; rather, the P_aCO_2 is increased because of the less than normal increase in $\dot{V}_E$, i.e., at any particular $\dot{V}_{CO_2}$; eqn (5.2). Consequently, CO_2 responsiveness as estimated from the standard CO_2-response curve (see Chapter 3) may be largely irrelevant to considerations of normal exercise hyperpnoea.

This lack of systematic change of mean P_aCO_2 and pH_a implies that it is highly unlikely that exercise hyperpnoea is under proportional, negative feedback control from such a stimulus. Consequently, other sources of stimulus – and of control – have been considered.

As described in Chapter 4, alterations in the dynamic features of the respiratory-related oscillations of P_aCO_2 and pH_a have been considered as the CO_2-linked stimulus. And while the rate of change, especially, of the oscillation is indeed related to the rate of pulmonary CO_2 exchange and has further been shown to influence $\dot{V}_E$, it is unlikely that these oscillations account for an appreciable component of the control – at best, it is the proportion of $\dot{V}_E$ decrement which results when the carotid bodies are 'silenced' by 100% O_2 being inhaled. And recently, the oscillations have been shown to be functionally eliminated as breathing frequency increases (to $20\,min^{-1}$, or even less) during exercise (Annastasiades *et al.*, 1985).

Other sources of carotid body stimulation may also be involved, such as the increase in arterial $[K^+]$ and osmolarity, but again are

Fig. 5.8 (opposite) Ventilatory and gas exchange responses to diversion of venous blood (between open arrows) during steady-state exercise (between solid arrows) in an anaesthetised dog. $\dot{V}_{exp}$, expiratory flow; P_{RV}, right ventricular blood pressure; BP, systemic arterial blood pressure; $\dot{Q}_{bypass}$, diverted blood flow. (From Huszczuk *et al.*, 1986*a*).

only likely to represent a small, and O_2-labile, component of the hyperpnoea. And furthermore, such mechanisms are clearly not obligatory for a 'normal' φ3 $\dot{V}_E$ response and thus P_aCO_2 and pH_a regulation; subjects who have had both carotid bodies surgically resected – but who had normal pulmonary function and blood gases at the time of the study – have a normal φ3 response (Wasserman *et al.*, 1975).

The search for sources of humoral stimulation and their manner of incorporation into the overall control scheme continues. The alternative approach is to consider the known sites of humoral control: the chemoreceptors.

The carotid bodies have been demonstrated to subserve the entire, or virtually entire, role of peripheral chemosensitivity in man (see Chapter 2). These structures are considered to be crucial for ventilatory responsiveness to both acute hypoxia and metabolic acidosis. It may also be readily demonstrated that the carotid chemoreceptors subserve an important role in the hyperpnoeic response to steady-state exercise. For example, the abrupt and surreptitious replacement of air as the inspirate with a humidified, hyperoxic gas evokes a clear transient fall of $\dot{V}_E$ whose nadir in man is normally some 15–20% of the steady-state exercise $\dot{V}_E$ in euoxia (Dejours, 1964; Stockley, 1978; Whipp & Wasserman, 1980; Griffiths *et al.*, 1986), resulting from suppression of carotid body afferent drive (see Chapter 2). Thus, $\dot{V}_E$ appears to be driven by peripheral chemoreceptor mechanisms. Based upon this technique, therefore, the carotid body contribution to the φ3 hyperpnoea has been estimated to be greater during moderate exercise (some 15–20%) than at rest (about 10–15%); the absolute magnitude, of course, being significantly greater. The $\dot{V}_E$ response to hypoxia has also been shown to be increased by exercise (Weil *et al.*, 1972.), using a progressive hypoxic test with isocapnia carefully maintained (see Chapter 2).

In contrast, during sustained O_2-breathing the φ3 $\dot{V}_E$ can be relatively normal, suggesting that other mechanisms (e.g. a lowering of cerebrospinal fluid pH consequent to decreased cerebral blood and a reduced buffering by hemoglobin) may offset the effects of carotid body inactivation on $\dot{V}_E$. Similarly, as discussed earlier, subjects whose carotid bodies have been surgically removed also display a reasonably normal φ3 hyperpnoea (Wasserman *et al.*, 1975). Again, this suggests that the role of the carotid bodies in φ3 control can be subsumed by other mechanisms; although, in this instance, it is unclear which mechanisms may be involved. An alternative explanation for this finding, however, is that the φ3 $\dot{V}_E$ was in fact reduced as a result of carotid body removal, but that previously a hyperventilatory component had existed (this is not uncommon in subjects with bronchial asthma, and the carotid body resected subjects who were investigated had this condition).

The most striking evidence of an important role of the carotid bodies in the hyperpnoea of moderate exercise can be found in the change in the φ2 $\dot{V}_E$ dynamics (Figure 5.7). If peripheral chemoreceptor gain is increased (e.g. by inhaling an hypoxic gas), the φ2 τ $\dot{V}_E$ is appreciably speeded; in contrast, hyperoxic mixtures slow the φ2 dynamics (see Cunningham, 1974; Casaburi *et al.*, 1980; Oren *et al.*, 1982; Griffiths *et al.*, 1986) and delays its onset (see Cunningham, 1974). For values of F_IO_2 (the inhaled oxygen fraction) of 12%–100% (which resulted in carotid body contributions to the total $\dot{V}_E$ drive ranging from some 50% with 12% O_2 to zero with hyperoxia), $\tau\dot{V}_E$ can change fourfold – from less than 30 s to some 2 min (Griffiths *et al.*, 1986). Dynamic $\dot{V}_E$ responses associated with sustained metabolic acidosis, which also increases peripheral chemoreceptor gain, provide further support for this concept (Oren *et al.*, 1982). Importantly, with respect to control dynamics, the response maintains its exponentiality over this wide range of carotid body drive. Furthermore, when peripheral chemoreceptor gain is reduced pharmacologically by the intravenous infusion of dopamine, $\tau\dot{V}_E$ is slowed (Boetger & Ward, 1985). And finally, subjects who had had both carotid bodies resected but who (at the time of the study) had normal pulmonary mechanics and blood gases, also responded to a square-wave exercise bout with a $\dot{V}_E$ time course that was appreciably slower than for control subjects (Wasserman *et al.*, 1976).

The systematic reduction of $\tau\dot{V}_E$ with increased carotid body gain has an important functional implication. As the hypoxaemia which occurs during φ2 in response to square-wave exercise, even in normal subjects, is a consequence of the ratio $\tau\dot{V}_E/\tau\dot{V}_{O_2}$ being appreciably greater than unity, then the reduction of $\tau\dot{V}_E$ under hypoxic conditions (e.g., at altitude or with hypoxaemia-inducing pulmonary disease) will constrain any further hypoxaemia during the transient.

Above θ_{an}, it appears in man that the compensatory hyperventilation for the metabolic acidosis of supra-θ_{an} exercise is mediated largely, if not exclusively, by the carotid bodies. Inactivation of these organs either by surgical resection (Wasserman *et al.*, 1975) or by O_2-breathing (Asmussen & Nielsen, 1958; Wilson & Welch, 1975) largely or completely abolishes the respiratory compensation for the metabolic acidosis (Wasserman *et al.*, 1975; Whipp & Wasserman, 1980; Figure 5.5). Consequently, pH_a falls more for a given $[HCO_3^-]_a$ decrease, and P_aCO_2 can actually be higher than the sub-θ_{an} exercise level – owing to the lack of, the reduced, or the slowed response to H^+ ions in the phase of the increased CO_2 load from the acid buffering.

Central chemoreceptor mechanisms, on the other hand, appear not to have an important role in the control of exercise hyperpnoea. This conclusion is based upon failure to discern a recognisable stimulus in the cerebrospinal fluid (c.s.f.) in the steady state (Leusen *et al.*, 1965; Bisgard *et al.*, 1978). Although it has not been possible to determine the acid-base characteristics of the brain extracellular fluid in the chemosensory region during exercise, it should be noted that the composition of bulk c.s.f. can be quite misleading in this respect especially during transients. Millhorn *et al.* (1984) were able to discern a small respiratory-related fluctuation in pH transmitted to brain extracellular fluid (adjacent to the medullary chemosensory regions) from the corresponding P_aCO_2 oscillations in the cat; no $\dot{V}_E$ response was evident, however. In contrast, Spode & Schlaefke (1975) have reported that blocking the 'intermediate' area on the ventral medullary surface actually abolished exercise hyperpnoea in peripherally deafferented cats. This suggests either that central chemoreceptor afferents (postulated to course through the intermediate area) do play a significant role in $\dot{V}_E$ control during exercise or that some other afferent excitatory influence can be inhibited by this regional block. This interesting possibility awaits further experimental consideration.

As described in this review, numerous afferent drives to the respiratory neural network in the brainstem have been documented experimentally and several competing control schemes proposed which range between predominantly neural and predominantly humoral control. However, it should be recognised that the demonstration of one mechanism being operative – in a given condition – does not rule out the potential for one or more of the others also to be operative. Consequently, the appropriate question with regard to exercise hyperpnoea (considering the spectrum of documented inputs) may not be why does ventilation increase, but rather why – for moderate exercise – does it normally only increase to levels commensurate with the level of CO_2 exchange?

5.5 **Further reading**

Dejours, P. (1964). Control of respiration in muscular exercise. In: *Handbook of Physiology*, (Fenn, W. O. & Rahn, H., eds.), pp. 631–48. American Physiological Society, Washington, D.C.

Dempsey, J. A., Mitchell, G. S. & Smith, C. A. (1984). Exercise and chemoreception. *American Review of Respiratory Disease*, **129**, 31–4.

Eldridge, F. L., Millhorn, D. E., Kiley, J. P. & Waldrop, T. G. (1985). Stimulation by central command of locomotion, respiration and circulation during exercise. *Respiration Physiology*, **59**, 313–37.

Kao, F. F. (1963). An experimental study of the pathways involved in exercise hyperpnea employing cross-circulation techniques. In: *The Regulation of Human Respiration*, (Cunningham, D. J. C. & Lloyd, B. B., eds.), pp. 461–502. Blackwell, Oxford.

Wasserman, K., Whipp, B. J. & Casaburi, R. (1986). Respiratory control during exercise. In: *Handbook of Physiology. The Respiratory System, II*, (Cherniack, N. S. & Widdicombe, J. G., eds.), pp. 595–619. American Physiological Society, Washington, D.C.

Whipp, B. J. (1981). The control of exercise hyperpnea. In: *The Regulation of Breathing*, (Hornbein, T., ed.), pp. 1069–139. Dekker, New York.

References

Adams, L., Frankel, H., Garlick, J., Guz, A., Murphy, K. & Semple, S. J. G. (1984). The role of spinal cord transmission in the ventilatory response to exercise in man. *Journal of Physiology*, **355**, 85–97.

Annastasiades, E., Cross, B. A., Guz, A., Leaver, K. D., Murphy, K., Phillips, M., Semple, S. J. G. & Stidwell, R. P. (1985). Continuous arterial pH measurement during exercise in patients with arteriovenous shunts. *Proceedings of the Physiological Society* September, 161P.

Asmussen, E., Johansen, S. H., Jorgensen, M. & Nielsen, M. (1965). On the nervous factors controlling respiration and circulation during exercise. *Acta Physiologica Scandinavica*, **63**, 343–50.

Asmussen, E. & Nielsen, M. (1958). Pulmonary ventilation and effect of oxygen breathing in heavy exercise. *Acta Physiologica Scandinavica*, **43**, 365–78.

Asmussen, E., Nielsen, M. & Wieth-Pedersen, G. (1943). Cortical or reflex control of respiration during muscular work? *Acta Physiologica Scandinavica*, **6**, 168–75.

Band, D. M., Linton, R. A. F., Kent, R. & Kurer, F. L. (1985). The effect of peripheral chemodenervation on the ventilatory response to potassium. *Respiration Physiology*, **60**, 217–25.

Bisgard, G. E., Forster, H. V., Byrnes, B., Stanek, K., Klein, J. & Manohar, M. (1978). Cerebrospinal fluid acid-base balance during muscular exercise. *Journal of Applied Physiology*, **45**, 94–101.

Boetger, C. L. & Ward, D. S. (1985). The effect of dopamine on the exercise hyperpnea. *Federation Proceedings*, **44**, 832.

Brice, G., Forster, H. V., Pan, L., Funahashi, M., Hoffman, T., Lowry, T. & Murphy, C. (1986). Is the hyperpnea during electrically-induced exercise (Ex_E) critically dependent on spinal afferents? *Federation Proceedings*, **45**, 518.

Casaburi, R., Stremel, R. W., Whipp, B. J., Beaver, W. L. & Wasserman, K. (1980). Alteration by hyperoxia of ventilatory dynamics during sinusoidal work. *Journal of Applied Physiology*, **48**, 1083–91.

Casaburi, R., Whipp, B. J., Wasserman, K., Beaver, W. L. & Koyal, S. N. (1977). Ventilatory and gas exchange dynamics in response to sinusoidal work. *Journal of Applied Physiology*, **42**, 300–11.

Cross, B. A., Davey, A., Guz, A., Katona, P. G., Maclean, M., Murphy, K., Semple, S. J. G. & Stidwell, R. (1982). The role of spinal cord transmission in the ventilatory response to electrically induced exercise in the anaesthetized dog. *Journal of Physiology*, **329**, 37–55.

Cunningham, D. J. C. (1974). Integrative aspects of the regulation of breathing; a personal view. In: *MTP International Review of Scientific Physiology* (Widdcombe, J. G., ed.) pp. 303–69. Butterworths, London.

Daly, W. J. & Overly, T. (1966). Modification of ventilatory regulation by hypnosis. *Journal of Laboratory and Clinical Medicine*, **68**, 279–85.

Dejours, P. (1964). Control of respiration in muscular exercise. In: *Handbook of Physiology* (Fenn, W. O. & Rahn, H., eds.), pp. 631–48. American Physiological Society, Washington, D.C.

Dejours, P., Labrousse, Y. & Teillac, A. (1959). Etude du stimulus ventilatoire proprioceptif mis en jeu par l'activite motrice chez l'homme. *Comptes Rendus de l'Acadamie des Sciences*, **248**, 2129–31.

Dempsey, J. A., Mitchell, G. S. & Smith, C. A. (1984). Exercise and chemoreception. *American Review of Respiratory Disease*, **129**, 31–4.

Eldridge, F. L. (1977). Maintenance of respiration by central neural feedback mechanisms. *Federation Proceedings*, **36**, 2400–4.

Eldridge, F. L., Millhorn, D. E., Kiley, J. P. & Waldrop, T. G. (1985). Stimulation by central command of locomotion, respiration and circulation during exercise. *Respiration Physiology*, **59**, 313–37.

Fordyce, W. E. & Bennett, F. M. (1984). Some characteristics of a steady state model of exercise hyperpnea. *Physiologist*, **27**, 217.

Goodwin, G. M., McCloskey, D. I. & Mitchell, J. H. (1972). Cardiovascular and respiratory responses to changes in central command during isometric exercise at constant muscle tension. *Journal of Physiology*, **226**, 173–90.

Green, J. F. & Sheldon, M. I. (1983). Ventilatory changes associated with changes in pulmonary blood flow in dogs. *Journal of Applied Physiology*, **54**, 997–1002.

Griffiths, T. L., Henson, L. C. & Whipp, B. J. (1986). The influence of inspired O_2 concentration on the dynamics of the exercise hyperpnoea in man. *Journal of Physiology*, **380**, 387–403.

Hagberg, J. M., Coyle, E. F., Carroll, J. E., Miller, J. M., Martin, W. H. & Brooke, M. H. (1982). Exercise hyperventilation in patients with McArdle's disease. *Journal of Applied Physiology*, **52**, 991–4.

Hodgson, H. J. F. & Mathews, P. B. C. (1968). The ineffectiveness of excitation of the primary endings of the muscle spindle by vibration as a respiratory stimulant in the decerbrate cat. *Journal of Physiology*, **194**, 555–63.

Huszczuk, A., Jones, P. W., Oren, A., Shors, E. C., Nery, L. E., Whipp, B. J. & Wasserman, K. (1983). Venous return and ventilatory control. In: *Modelling and Control of Breathing* (Whipp, B. J. & Wiberg, D. M., eds.) pp. 78–85. Elsevier, New York.

Huszczuk, A., Whipp, B. J., Oren, A., Shors, E. C., Pokorski, M., Nery, L. E. & Wasserman, K. (1986*a*). Ventilatory responses to partial cardiopulmonary bypass at rest and during exercise in dogs. *Journal of Applied Physiology*, **61**, 575–83.

Huszczuk, A., Whipp, B. J., Wasserman, K., Adams, T. D., Fisher, A. G., Olsen, D. B., Crapo, R. O. & Elliott, C. G. (1986*b*). Ventilatory control during exercise in calves with artificial (Jarvick) hearts. *Federation Proceedings*, **45**, 1127.

Jensen, J. I. (1972). Neural ventilatory drive during arm and leg exercise. *Scandinavian Journal of Clinical and Laboratory Investigation*, **29**, 117–84.

Jones, N. L. (1975). Exercise testing in pulmonary evaluation: rationale, methods, and the normal respiratory response to exercise. *New England Journal of Medicine*, **293**, 541–4.

Jones, N. L. & Haddon, R. W. T. (1973). Effect of a meal on cardiopulmonary and metabolic changes during exercise. *Canadian Journal of Physiology and Pharmacology*, **51**, 445–50.

Jones, P. W., French, W., Weissman, M. L. & Wasserman, K. (1981). Ventilatory responses to cardiac output changes in patients with pacemakers. *Journal of Applied Physiology*, **51**, 1103–7.

Jones, P. W., Huszczuk, A. & Wasserman, K. (1982). Cardiac output as a controller of ventilation through changes in right ventricular load. *Journal of Applied Physiology*, **53**, 218–44.

Kao, F. F. (1963). An experimental study of the pathways involved in exercise hyperpnea employing cross-circulation techniques. In: *The Regulation of Human Respiration*, (Cunningham, D. J. C. & Lloyd, B. B., eds.) pp. 461–502. Blackwell, Oxford.

Karlsson, H., Lindborg, B. & Linnarsson, D. (1975). Time courses of pulmonary gas exchange and heart rate changes in supine exercise. *Acta Physiologica Scandinavica*, **95**, 329–40.

Kostreva, D. R., Zuperku, E. J., Purtock, R. V., Coon, R. L. & Kampine, J. P. (1975). Sympathetic afferent nerve activity of right heart origin. *American Journal of Physiology*, **229**, 911–15.

Krogh, A. & Lindhard, J. (1913). The regulation of respiration and circulation during the initial stages of muscular work. *Journal of Physiology*, **47**, 112–36.

Leusen, I. (1965). Aspects of the acid-base balance between blood and cerebrospinal fluid. In: *Cerebrospinal Fluid and the Regulation of Ventilation*, (Brooks, C., Kao, F. F. & Lloyd, B. B., eds.) pp. 55–89. Blackwell, Oxford.

Levine, S. (1978). Stimulation of ventilation by exercise-released humoral agents: Role of extra-cranial receptors. *Chest*, **73**, 279–80.

Lloyd, T. C. Jr (1984). Effect on breathing of acute pressure rise in pulmonary artery and right ventricle. *Journal of Applied Physiology*, **57**, 110–16.

McCloskey, E. I. & Mitchell, J. H. (1972). Reflex cardiovascular and respiratory responses originating in exercising muscle. *Journal of Physiology*, **224**, 173–86.

Millhorn, D. E., Eldridge, F. L. & Kiley, J. P. (1984). Oscillation of medullary extracellular fluid pH caused by breathing. *Respiration Physiology*, **55**, 193–203.

Morgan, W. P., Raven, P. B., Drinkwater, B. L. & Horvath, S. M. (1973). Perceptual and metabolic responsivity to standard bicycle ergometry following various hypnotic suggestions. *International Journal of Clinical and Experimental Hypnosis*, **21**, 86–101.

Oldenburg, F. A., McCormack, D. W., Morse, J. L. C. & Jones, N. L. (1979). A comparison of exercise responses in stairclimbing and cycling. *Journal of Applied Physiology*, **46**, 510–16.

Oren, A., Wasserman, K., Davis, J. A. & Whipp, B. J. (1981). The effect of CO_2 set-point on the ventilatory response to exercise. *Journal of Applied Physiology*, **51**, 185–9.

Oren, A., Whipp, B. J. & Wasserman, K. (1982). Effect of acid-base status on the kinetics of the ventilatory response to moderate exercise. *Journal of Applied Physiology*, **52**, 1013–17.

Poon, C. S. (1983). Optimal control of ventilation in hypoxia, hypercapnia and exercise. In: *Modeling and Control of Breathing* (Whipp, B. J. & Wiberg, D. M., eds.) pp. 189–96. Elsevier, New York.

Spode, R. & Schlaefke, M. E. (1975). Influence of muscular exercise on respiration after central and peripheral denervation. *Pflugers Archives* suppl. 359, R49.

Stockley, R. A. (1978). The contribution of the reflex hypoxic drive to the hyperpnoea of exercise. *Respiration Physiology*, **35**, 79–87.

Theodore, J., Robin, E. D., Morris, A. J. R., Burke, C. M., Jamieson, S. W., Van Kessel, A., Stinson, E. B. & Shumway, N. E. (1986). Augmented ventilatory response to exercise in pulmonary hypertension. *Chest*, **89**, 39–44.

Tibes, U. (1977). Reflex inputs to the cardiovascular and respiratory centers from dynamically working canine muscles. *Circulation Respiration*, **41**, 332–431.

Trenchard, D. (1986). Confirmation of chemosensitivity of 'pulmonary' endings by use of a differential vagal nerve block in anaesthetized rabbits. *Proceedings of the Physiological Society* February, 58P.

Uchida, Y. (1986). Tachypnea after stimulation of afferent cardiac sympathetic nerve fibres. *American Journal of Physiology*, **230**, 1003–7.

Wasserman, K. & Mcilroy, M. B. (1964). Detecting the threshold of anaerobic metabolism. *American Journal of Cardiology*, **14**, 844–52.

Wasserman, K., Van Kessel, A. L. & Burton, G. G. (1967). Interaction of physiological mechanisms during exercise. *Journal of Applied Physiology*, **22**, 71–85.

Wasserman, K., Whipp, B. J., Casaburi, R., Beaver, W. L. & Brown, H. F. (1977). CO_2 flow to the lungs and ventilatory control. In: *Muscular Exercise and the Lungs* (Dempsey, J. A. & Reed, C. E., eds.) pp. 103–35. University of Wisconsin Press, Madison.

Wasserman, K., Whipp, B. J. & Castagna, J. (1974). Cardiodynamic hyperpnea: hyperpnea secondary to cardiac output increase. *Journal of Applied Physiology*, **36**, 457–64.

Wasserman, K., Whipp, B. J., Koyal, S. N. & Cleary, M. G. (1975). Effect of carotid body resection on ventilatory and acid-base control during exercise. *Journal of Applied Physiology*, **39**, 354–8.

Weil, J. V., Byrne-Quinn, E., Sodal, I. E., Kline, J. E., McCullough, R. E. & Filley, G. F. (1972). Augmentation of chemosensitivity during mild exercise in normal man. *Journal of Applied Physiology*, **33**, 813–19.

Weiler-Ravell, D., Cooper, D. M., Whipp, B. J. & Wasserman, K. (1983). Control of breathing at the start of exercise as influenced by posture. *Journal of Applied Physiology*, **55**, 1460–6.

Weisman, M. L., Wasserman, K., Huntsman, D. J. & Whipp, B. J. (1979). Ventilation and gas exchange during phasic hindlimb exercise in the dog. *Journal of Applied Physiology*, **46**, 874–84.

Weissman, M. L., Jones, P. W., Oren, A., Lamarra, N., Whipp, B. J. &

Wasserman, K. (1982). Cardiac output increase and gas exchange at start of exercise. *Journal of Applied Physiology*, **52**, 236–44.

Whipp, B. J. (1977). The hyperpnoea of dynamic muscular exercise. In: *Exercise and Sport Science Reviews* (Hulton, R. S., ed.), pp. 295–311, Journal Publishing, Affiliates, Santa Barbara.

Whipp, B. J. (1981). The control of exercise hyperpnea. In: *The Regulation of Breathing* (Hornbein, T., ed.) pp. 1069–139. Dekker, New York.

Whipp, B. J. & Pardy, R. L. (1986). Breathing diving exercise. In: *Handbook of Physiology Section 3 The Respiratory System*, Vol. 3, pp. 605–29 (Cherniak, N. S. & Widdicombe, J. G., eds.), The American Physiological Society, Washington D.C.

Whipp, B. J. & Ward, S. A. (1980). Ventilatory central dynamics during muscular exercise in man. *International Journal of Sports Medicine*, **1**, 146–59.

Whipp, B. J. & Ward, S. A. (1982). Cardiopulmonary coupling during exercise. *Journal of Experimental Biology*, **100**, 175–93.

Whipp, B. J. & Ward, S. A. (1985). Cardio pulmonary system responses to muscular exercise in man. In: *Circulation, Respiration and Metabolism* (Gilles, R., ed.), pp. 64–80, Springer, Berlin.

Whipp, B. J. & Wasserman, K. (1980). Carotid bodies and ventilatory control dynamics in man. *Federation Proceedings*, **39**, 2628–73.

Wilson, H. D. & Welch, H. G. (1975). Effects of hyperoxic gas mixtures on exercise tolerance in man. *Medicine and Science in Sports*, **7**, 48–52.

Young, I. H. & Woolcock, A. J. (1978). Changes in arterial blood gas tensions during unsteady-state exercise. *Journal of Applied Physiology*, **44**, 93–6.

Index

air flow
  'choke point' 10
  limitation 10
  maximum flow-volume 8, 10
  maximum wave speed 10
  mean expiratory 2
  mean inspiratory 2
  patterns 1, 2, 6
  resistance 12, 22
  spontaneous flow-volume 8
alveolar PCO_2
  breath-to-breath alternations 17
  time profile 17, 50, 51
  within-breath oscillation 48, 50, 51
apnea 14
apneusis 19
artificial (Jarvik) heart and exercise hyperpnoea 107

breathing
  breathing-by-breath variability 2
breathing pattern 2, 10, 11, 53
  blood gas regulation (exercise) 88, 96
  breathing apparatus 23, 24, 54, 55
  bronchoconstriction 13
  cardiopulmonary bypass 14
  expiratory braking 19
  expiratory-inspiratory switching 20
  FRC 10, 11
  hypercapnia 16
  hypoxia 16
  inspiratory 'duty cycle' 21
  inspiratory off-switch 18
  timing of stimulus 72
  vagotomy 14
bronchoconstriction
  influence on breathing pattern 13

carbon dioxide
  alveolar 17, 45
  arterial regulation 89, 94, 95, 98, 107
  responsiveness 39
  role in breathing pattern 16
carbon dioxide response curve
  constant flow 47, 61
  exercise 46, 47, 60, 61, 62
  hypoxia 53
  oscillations of partial pressure 68, 69, 109
  rebreathing 47, 48, 53, 60, 61
carbonic anhydrase 70
cardiac transplantation and exercise hyperpnoea 107
cardiodynamic hyperpnea 106
cardiopulmonary bypass 14, 106, 107
cardiopulmonary coupling 82, 102, 104
carotid bodies
  hypoxia 29, 30
  PCO_2, pH oscillation 70, 71, 72, 73, 75, 76, 109
carotid body resection 32, 41, 110, 111
carotid endarterectomy 32
catecholamines
  modulation of hypoxic responsiveness 39

centrally-generated inspiratory activity (CIA) 18, 19
cerebral perfusion
effect of superior cervical ganglionectomy 85
hypercapnia 55
hypoxia 36
chemoreceptors
arterial 15, 17, 29, 49, 50, 58, 103, 112
central (medullary) 15, 49, 50, 56, 58, 103
compliance
lung 22
respiratory system 11, 12
cortical irradiation 80, 104

dead space 89, 90
diaphragm
blood flow 23
EMG 21, 22
efficiency 22
domains of exercise
intensity 88
temporal 87

electromyography 4
end-expiratory lung volume 1
exercise
breathing following spinal cord transection 78, 80, 104
electrically-induced 78, 80
hyperpnoea 78–82, 87–113
influence on breathing pattern 6
modulation of hypoxic responsiveness 39

flow-volume curves
maximal 8, 10
spontaneous 8
functional residual capacity 1, 10
influence on mouth occlusion pressure 22

gas stores of body
influence on O_2 uptake and CO_2 kinetics during exercise 102
glomus pulmonale 32

Hering–Breuer inflation reflex 5, 13
hyperpnoea of exercise *see* exercise hyperpnoea
hypnotic suggestion and exercise hyperpnoea 105
hypothalamic motor area 105
hypoxia
altitude 29
assessment 40, 41
carotid bodies 29, 32, 33
influence on breathing pattern 6
influence on cerebral metabolic acidosis 33
influence on cerebral perfusion 36
sensitivity 30, 31
modulators of ventilatory response 30, 31, 40, 41, 110
parameters 40
stimulus pattern 38
ventilatory depression 33, 37, 40

ideal lung 88
impulse-function (or short 'pulse')
exercise stimulus 99
hypercapnic stimulus 52
hypoxic stimulus 38
'intermediate area (ventral medulla) and exercise hyperpnoea 112
isocapnic breathing 6

'J' Receptors *see* receptors

kinetics of ventilation and gas exchange during exercise 99, 100, 101, 102, 110, 111

lactic acid
buffering by bicarbonate system 92
intensity domains of exercise 88
larynx
influence on airway resistance 12
locomotor centre (sub-hypothalamic) 80, 105
locomotor-ventilatory coupling 80, 105

muscle reflexogenic drive (exercise) 103
muscle spindles and exercise hyperpnoea 103
muscles of breathing
abdominals 4, 19, 80
diaphragm: EMG 21, 11
efficiency 22
intercostals 22, 80
laryngeal abductor 12
posterior cricoarytaenoid 12, 20

nerve fibres
gamma afferents and exercise hyperpnoea 104
groups III and IV and exercise hyperpnoea 103
myelinated fibres and exercise hyperpnoea 103
unmyelinated 'c' type 13, 14
nerves
phrenic
electroneurogram 21, 22, 52, 72
vagus
effect of cooling 13
nose-clip
influence on breathing pattern 23, 54, 55

optimisation of respiratory work 23
oscillations
arterial PCO_2 (pH) 48, 50, 51, 68, 69, 109

pattern of breathing *see* breathing pattern
pressure
intra-thoracic 13
physiological dead-space 89, 90
pulmonary circulatory transit times 38

ramp function
exercise stimulus 99
hypoxic stimulus 38
receptors
CO_2-sensitive (birds and lizards)14
irritant 13
juxta pulmonary capillary ('j') 14
rapidly-adapting 13, 19
slowly-adapting stretch 13, 14, 20
reflex
Head's paradoxical 13
Hering–Breur inflation 5, 13
resistance
airway 22, 24
expiratory (non-elastic) 10
influence of larynx 19
respiratory centres 1, 18
nucleus parabrachialis medialis (NPBM) 18, 19
pneumotoxic 18, 19
pontomedullary 72, 80
respiratory compensation for metabolic acidosis 95, 98, 112
respiratory work 1, 22, 23
optimisation 23
reverberation (neural) and exercise hyperpnoea 105
right-ventricular pressure and exercise hyperpnoea 106

set point for PCO_2 89

sinusoidal function
  exercise stimulus 99
  hypercapnic stimulus 49
  hypoxic stimulus 38
step-function
  exercise stimulus 99
  hypercapnic stimulus 49, 58
  hypoxic stimulus 38
superior cervical ganglionectomy
  influence on brainstem blood flow 55
sympathetic afferents (cardiac and exercise hyperpnoea) 106

temperature
  influence on breathing pattern 6
  influence on inspiratory off-switch 19
  modulation of hypoxic responsiveness 39
time constant
  mechanical (of respiratory system) 12
timing effect
  relationship between time of stimulus and phase of respiratory cycle 17, 18, 69, 72, 73

vagotomy
  apneusis 19
  effect on pattern of breathing 14

ventilation
  alveolar 88, 89, 93
  minute 1
  response to exercise 78–82, 87–113
  response to hypoxia 30, 31, 32, 40, 41

ventilatory depression
  influence of hypoxia 33, 37, 40
ventilatory equivalent for CO_2 92, 104

work of breathing 1, 22, 23
  elastic 1
  minimum 23
  optimisation 23
  resistive 1